Beat *the* Gym

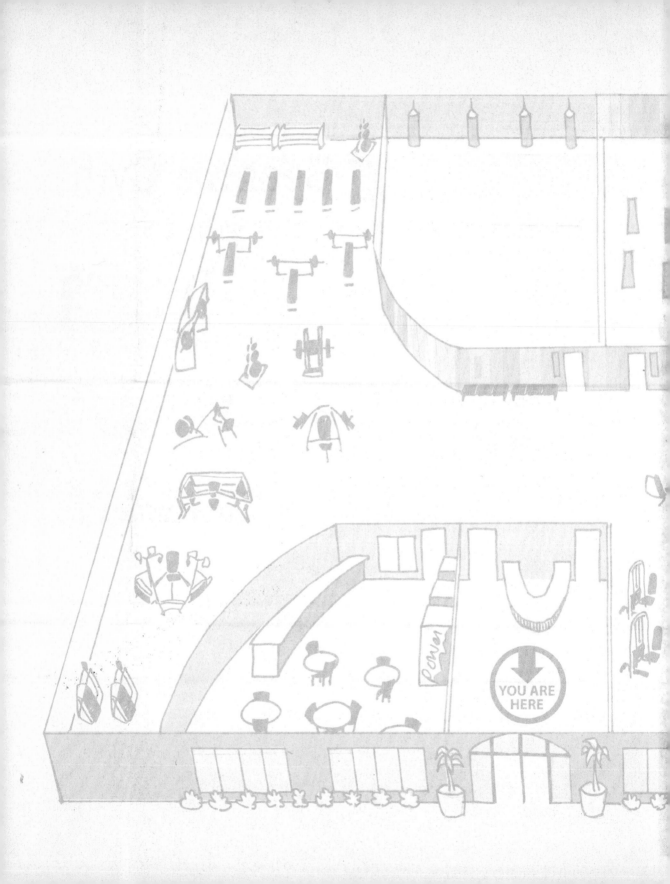

Beat *the* Gym

Personal Trainer Secrets—Without the Personal Trainer Price Tag

TOM HOLLAND WITH MEGAN McMORRIS

WM

WILLIAM MORROW

An Imprint of HarperCollins*Publishers*

Photographs by Philippa Holland

HarperCollins books may be purchased for educational, business, or sales promotional use. For information please write: Special Markets Department, HarperCollins Publishers, 10 East 53rd Street, New York, NY 10022.

FIRST EDITION

Designed by Richard Oriolo

Library of Congress Cataloging-in-Publication Data

Holland, Tom.
    Beat the gym : personal trainer secrets—without the personal trainer price tag / Tom Holland with Megan McMorris. —1st ed.
      p. cm.
    ISBN 978-0-06-198405-1
  1. Exercise. 2. Physical fitness. 3. Health. I. McMorris, Megan. II. Title.
    GV481.H725 2011
    613.7—dc22

                      2010035176

11 12 13 14 15 ov/QG 10 9 8 7 6 5 4 3 2 1

This book is dedicated to my wife, Philippa,
and Thing One and Thing Two, my boys Tommy and Cooper

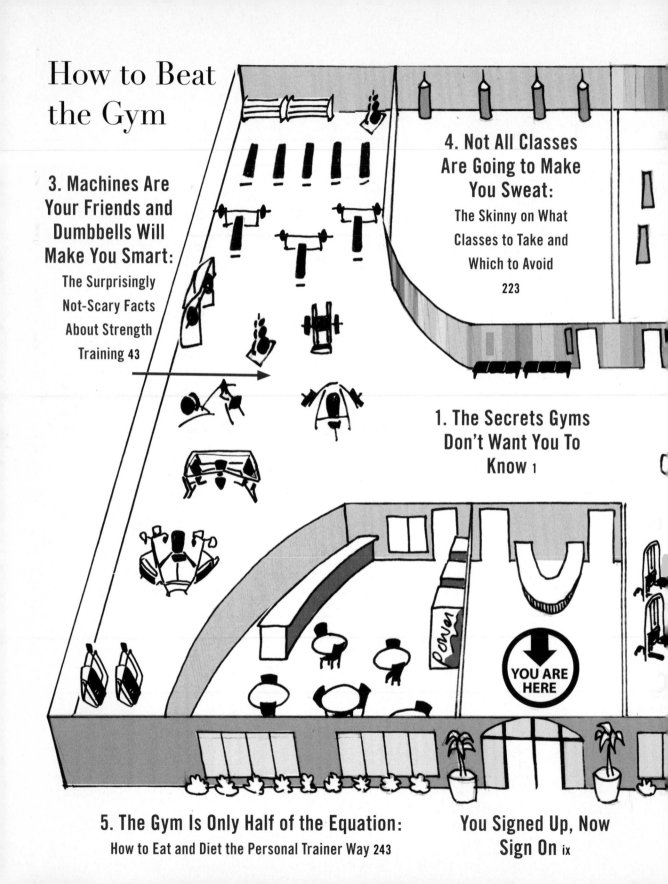

How to Beat the Gym

YOU ARE HERE

Power

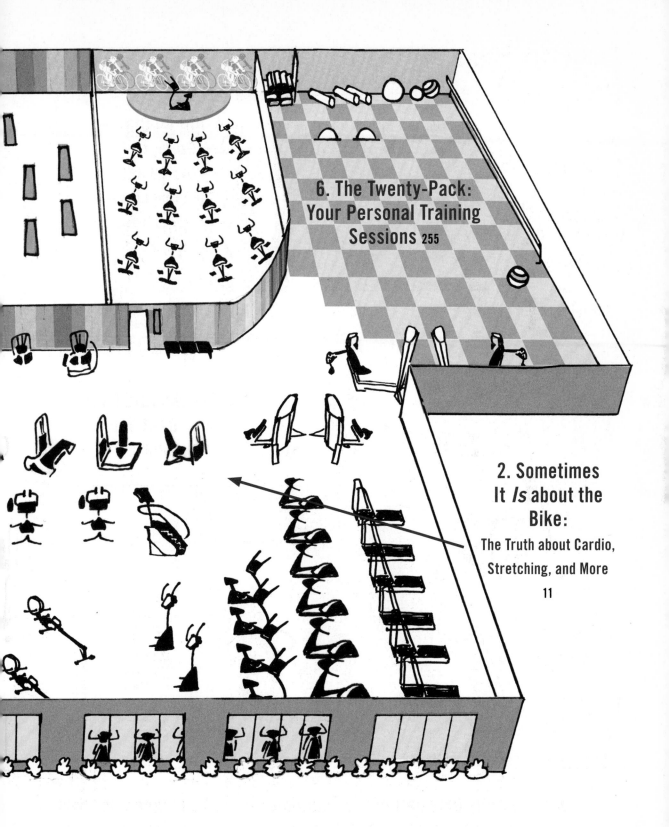

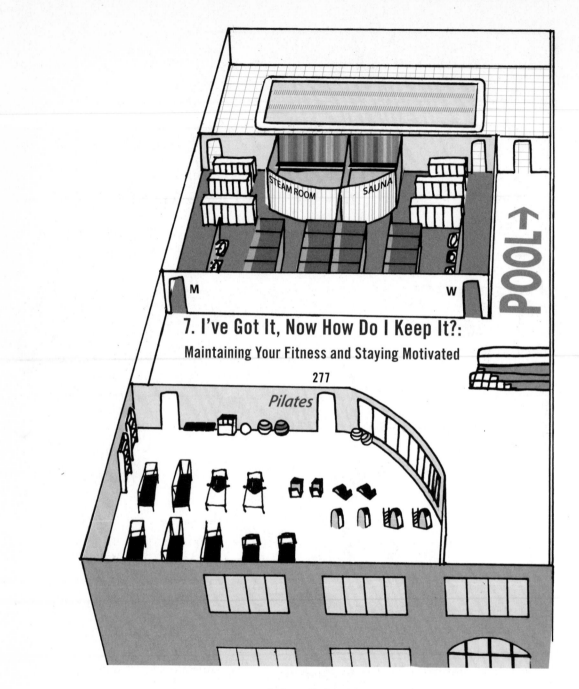

7. I've Got It, Now How Do I Keep It?:

Maintaining Your Fitness and Staying Motivated

277

You Signed Up, Now Sign On

You have invested hours of your time and a significant amount of money in your gym membership and workouts but have yet to see a big return on your investment. But don't beat yourself up; instead, BEAT THE GYM.

I have worked in the fitness industry for almost two decades now, first as a personal trainer at many of New York City's top gyms, then as a fitness instructor for elite athletes and celebrities, and now as the owner of my own gym, the Tom Holland Athletic Club in New Canaan, Connecticut; and I know that the big bad secret of seeing results is having a personal trainer provide you with a personalized workout and stand next you to motivate you to get it done. But personal trainers are incredibly expensive, and often it is difficult to find the right one. What I have set out to do in this book is give you the advice, training sessions, and support that are unique to the personal trainer experience so you will have the motivation and knowledge to finally reach your fitness goals.

I am here to be your personal trainer. I am here to help you look better, feel better, and, best of all, live longer. I have worked with thousands of people around the world to achieve all of the above, and I can help you do so as well. The best part is, it makes no difference which of the three is the reason you first decided to join a gym and start working out, you get all three.

But it's not that easy.

More than 60 percent of people who join a gym never return after three months. If you're like most people, you joined the gym with the best of intentions, all fired up and ready to change your body and your life, but so far all you have ended up with is frustration. I know how you feel; I see it every day at my own gym. It drives me crazy to watch people work out in vain. Members who have paid good money for their gym memberships take the time to show up and work out, yet they see few to no results. That really stinks. I often return to my old clubs in New York City and see the same people doing the same routines, looking *exactly the same as they did years ago.* They show up and work out three, four, five times a week but have literally nothing to show for their efforts. That's not okay. I want you to enjoy going to the gym and be committed and passionate about the workout. The way to do that is to be knowledgeable about what the gym truly offers and how you can make it work for you. How you can BEAT THE GYM.

I have the greatest job in the world, and I am in the unique position of being able to help you to look better, feel better, and live longer. There is nothing I enjoy more. That's why I have made that endeavor my life's work. I have both worked in and worked out in every type of gym imaginable. I spent years grinding away as a trainer and group fitness instructor in New York City, seven days a week, often seventeen-hour days. Crunch. Sports Club LA. Reebok. Equinox. New York Sports Clubs. The Cardio Fitness Center. Private homes and private gyms. Celebrities, CEOs, real people, I have shaped every body type imaginable. And I can transform yours.

At the same time as I was working my butt off as a trainer, I also set out to learn as much as I could about fitness. I have been certified by all of the top fitness organizations: the American College of Sports Medicine, the National Strength and Conditioning Association, the National Academy of Sports Medicine, the American Council on Exercise, and the Aerobics and Fitness Association of America. I went back to get a master's degree, not only in exercise science but with a concentration in sports psychology as well. After working with hundreds and hundreds of private clients I realized how important the mind is to this whole process of getting in shape.

Everyone is different; we all have different body types, different fitness histories, different personalities, different likes and dislikes, different schedules, and different goals.

So this book has many different plans. Should you do cardio or weights first? What's the best exercise to get a flat stomach? Are you a guy who wants bigger arms? Do you want to get the most out of your cardio workouts? Do you have an event you need to drop weight quickly for?

I also answer many of the most common questions you have when it comes to the gym: What classes should I take based on my goals? Do I need a trainer, and, if so, how do I go about choosing one? Which are better, free weights or machines? What should I eat before a workout? And after? After I achieve the body I want, how can I keep it? If I want a home gym, what equipment should I buy and why? I answer all these questions and many more. *You signed up, now sign on.* It is time to BEAT THE GYM. I have to warn you, I may come across a little strong in certain parts of the book. A little harsh, even. Just remember that I have your best intentions in mind. I want you to succeed. I know that you can. It's just that I get frustrated with all the misinformation out there that is keeping you from attaining your goals.

Beat the Gym is your road map to getting the most out of your workout. The most out of your gym membership. As I tell all my clients, you are now my advertising. I have a vested interest in your looking great, feeling great, and living longer. No more wasted time and wasted money. Today is the first day of your new program, the one that will actually deliver results. Results that will last a lifetime!

1.

The Secrets Gyms Don't
Want You to Know

When I first started working as a trainer at one of the major clubs in New York City, my goal was to learn as much about the fitness club world as possible, not simply the personal training and group fitness side but every aspect of the operations of a fitness club.

One day, when I was a very wet-behind-the-ears personal trainer, I stopped to talk with the general manager, who was standing at the front desk running reports.

"Quick question: how do you know when to stop taking memberships?"

She continued to type on the computer without looking up.

"What do you mean?"

"You know, is there a formula for the size of the gym and how many members it can have? Like, ten thousand square feet means two thousand members or something like that?"

She looked up at me and laughed.

"You mean when do we 'cap' memberships? What is our cutoff number? There isn't one. It doesn't exist. We just sell, sell, sell."

She laughed again and resumed typing.

There is no formula. Fitness club salespeople make money based on sales. They have monthly goals to hit. All they want to do is get people in the door.

And they hope many don't come back in. *Ever.*

Think about it: if just 25 percent of all the members of a gym showed up all at the same time, there would be complete chaos. Mayhem. There would be long lines for every treadmill, elliptical trainer, and leg-press machine. This leads to Rule 1 about most gyms:

Rule 1: Gyms Hope You Sign Up but Never Show Up

It's absolutely true. Most gyms are actually selling you a membership, asking you to come and join the club, welcoming you with open arms and big smiles, yet they really don't ever want to ever see you again. You would be shocked to find out how many total members there are in your gym. There are hundreds, sometimes thousands, of people at every fitness club who literally join, go a handful of times, then never step through the doors again. Ever. A huge percentage continue to have their credit cards billed month after month, often year after year.

Gym owners love those members.

Of the fraction who do use the gym, there exists an even smaller fraction who are referred to by management as the "heavy users." You know who these people are. You may even be one of them. The so-called hard-core members. They are the ones who do use the gym four, five, six days a week. Sometimes twice a day. They are getting the most for their money. If you are already one of those people, great. This book will help you take your workout to an even higher level.

Chances are, however, if you are reading this book, you are not one of these regular users. You are sporadic. You are like the majority of gym members: after New Year's, just before summer, those are the times you go to the gym. Then, inevitably, you fall off. Days, weeks, maybe even months go by without a single visit.

It all really comes down to motivation and incentive. Who can be motivated when putting in effort and getting nothing back? When you see results, you suddenly become motivated. Funny how that works. This book will help you change your body in ways you only dreamed were possible, regardless of how frequently you use the gym now.

Rule 2: Listen to the Pitch, Then Walk Away

Remember that most salespeople, no matter what they say as they schmooze you around the facility, couldn't care less about whether you lose weight, bulk up, slim down, whatever. All they really care about is closing the deal. They have monthly goals to hit. They are also on commission. You represent dollar signs, not much else. Such is life.

So during your initial visit to the gym, sign nothing, no matter how great the deal seems to be. They'll throw in free personal training, massages or free months, offer to wash your car, anything to get you to join right away. Don't. The fact remains that when you walk out the door that offer will still be good, regardless of what the salesperson says. More important, the offer will quite often be made even better after you leave. That person knows you are interested. He or she wants your money. The first pitch is just the starting point.

Rule 3: Do Not Sign the Contract in the Gym

Take the contract home with you and read it carefully, word for word. There's lots of small print. Trust me.

Rule 4: Once You Do Sign Up, It's Really Hard to Break Up

Ever try to get out of your gym membership? It can be much worse than trying to end a bad relationship. Many gyms require things like a doctor's note or proof that you have moved hundreds of miles away before they will even consider terminating your membership. And when you do end your contract, you often have to pay for a few months more before you are truly free.

Have the salesperson explain what the exact terms of ending the contract are.

Trainer Tip: The initiation fee is negotiable.

Most gyms have a onetime initiation fee. It can range from a few to hundreds of dollars. This initiation fee is in addition to your monthly gym payments. Be aware that, at almost every gym, this fee is completely negotiable. Ever notice how around New Year's or just before summer, gyms start to advertise "$0 initiation fee"? Take advantage of this when joining a gym. Start by refusing to pay any initiation fee at all. None. It's pretty much up to you and your negotiation skills. If you can't get the salesperson to knock it out completely, try cutting it in half. If you don't get what you want, walk away. Most likely the salesperson will have taken down your contact information. If you walk away, chances are very good that you will receive a phone call from the salesperson, reducing the initiation fee or wiping it out completely.

The main payment you will make to the gym is the membership fee. You will most often have two options for payment, monthly or paid in full. Many people choose to have their credit card charged monthly because they don't want to shell out all the money up front. This is a choice you have to make. Realize that many gyms will offer you a discount, for instance 10 percent off the total membership price, if you pay all at once. So you can save some more money there. Another benefit of paying up front is that it makes "breaking up" with the gym a little less complicated. Yes, you are locked in for a year unless you move or have a medical reason for leaving, but at the end of the year the contract is up. You can choose to renew or not. You won't have the hassle of trying to stop the monthly charges as you would if you choose to have your credit card charged every month.

Ask a Trainer: So you can negotiate the initiation fee; can you also negotiate the monthly fee?

The short answer is "Maybe." You can always try. If the monthly fee is $75, you can ask to have five, maybe ten bucks knocked off per month, especially if you are joining with a spouse or other family members. This is much harder to do than for the initiation fee, but you have a shot.

Choosing a Gym: It's All about Location, Location, Location

I don't care how beautiful the gym is; if it's not close, you're not going to go. Period. Don't kid yourself into thinking otherwise. Most people just aren't disciplined and motivated enough to travel even ten extra minutes to get to the gym on a consistent basis. I don't care how nice the showers are or how new the equipment is, it's all about convenience. Sure, you might go to that beautiful club that's a little farther away than you wanted for a few weeks. But as work and life start to get in the way, that commute can start to really get annoying. Even five extra minutes can be a problem, especially when time is tight, like when you want to take classes in the morning before work. Find a gym as close to you as possible, either where you live or where you work, depending on when you will be using it.

You don't have to love it. You just have to like it. Then you will use it.

Trainer Tip: Choose a gym as close to you as possible.

OTHER QUESTIONS TO ASK

1. What are the hours? Does the gym open early enough and/or stay open late enough for you?

2. Can you go whenever you want, or is your rate for "nonpeak" hours only?

3. Does the gym offer towel service? And if so, is there a fee? (Yes, some gyms actually *charge* you to use a towel!)

4. If the gym offers classes, are they included or is there an additional fee for them? Some gyms have one price for use of the gym only, another for classes only, and a third for both. Some gyms charge for certain classes (usually the popular ones), while others are free. Be sure to clarify this beforehand.

5. Does the gym offer babysitting? If so, how much does it cost?

6. If the gym has other locations, can you use them all or does that involve an additional fee?

Rule 5: Take the Gym for a Test Drive

Joining a gym for a year is a big commitment. You can't really tell what it's truly like by just spending a few minutes walking around. You really should try it out before signing on the dotted line. Most gyms will offer you a few free day passes or a free week. Take advantage of this. You want to work out at your potential new club at all the different times you would be using it. What's it like at peak hours? Can you get on a treadmill when you want to, or are there long lines? What are the people like? Is it too hot? Too cold? Too crowded? Not crowded enough? Can you get into the classes you want? Use everything you would be using if you joined, including the showers. Also see what your commute to and from the gym is like. Rule out all surprises before you make the big commitment.

Trainer Tip: Many gyms offer their freebies online.

If you are considering joining a specific gym, check out their website first. Many gyms will have things like free passes and special offers posted on their sites. Free day passes, free weeks, free introductory training sessions, and more. You can often print them out and bring then in for your free trial or discounts.

Rule 6: The "Free" Orientation Is All About Selling You Personal Training

When you are sitting in front of the salesperson at a fitness club deciding whether or not you will join, he or she will inevitably start to list for you all the wonderful things that come with your membership in an effort to sweeten and ultimately close the deal. One of those incentives is usually a free personal training session. Or two, possibly even three sessions. While the salesperson may tell you that this session is a great way for you to learn how to use the equipment so that you can do it on your own, that's the exact opposite of what the club management wants. The sessions are in fact opportunities for trainers to show you how much you need them, how little you know, and how you can't possibly work out on your own. They are trained salesmen, taught the difference between open- and closed-ended questions. At the end of the session you will not be asked "So do you want to buy personal training sessions?" No, a seasoned trainer will take you through a fantastic workout, one that you can't possibly do on your own, then take you to the personal training desk and say "So, do you want to buy a twenty-pack or fifty-pack of personal training sessions?"

Why give two or three free training sessions? Is it pure altruism? Not quite. If the trainer can't sell you after the first time, it gives him or another trainer another chance to reel you in.

Trainer Tip: Most trainers will give you a free session.

All you have to do is ask. Trainers make their money by training clients. By approaching a trainer and asking for a workout, you are expressing that you are interested in working with that person and that you are a potential client. Most will welcome the opportunity to sell you what they're peddling. Take the trainer for a test drive. Give him or her a chance to "wow" you. If you like that person, you can buy a package. If not, move on to another trainer. Trainers are expensive. You can literally do a free session with every trainer in the gym if you want. Just because you don't have a free session from the gym doesn't mean you can't ask for one. Most gyms couldn't care less about letting a trainer do a free session. In fact, they often encourage it. It costs them nothing and holds the potential for the club to make money when the trainer converts you into a paying client.

But be warned: the free workout the trainer gives you is often designed for one specific purpose: to hook you in and get you to purchase personal training sessions. To make you believe that you can get the workout only with that trainer. That you cannot possibly do it alone. This is why the trainer rarely puts you on machines. The trainer will also avoid writing things down for you. He or she wants you to leave feeling that you got an amazing workout that you can't duplicate without working with the trainer.

Rule 7: The Salesperson Will Often Try to Sell You with Things That Won't Make You Any Fitter

What is the number one thing most people look for in a gym? Is it the latest equipment? Cutting-edge classes? A cheap monthly rate? Nope.

You know what ranks ridiculously high on the list of what people look for in a gym?

Cleanliness.

That's right. Clean equipment. Clean locker rooms. Nothing to do with what is going to really get you in shape.

So the gym owners know and exploit this fact. That's why when you get your introductory tour of the gym the salespeople don't spend too much time on the finer points of the exercise equipment. They show you the sparkling clean showers. The pristine changing room. They'll even make a point of taking you through the group exercise studio as the cleaning crew is mopping the floor.

They will sell you on everything but what will help you get in shape.

Many, many years ago I moved to New York City. I was fresh out of college and ready to try my hand at my numerous short-lived preexercise jobs. And I needed a gym to work out in. I walked into the club that was closest to my apartment, which happened also to be one of the "hottest" and most expensive at the time. The salesman spent almost no time explaining what the gym had to offer, but he did make a point of taking me to one particular section of the gym. There was a class going on, and it was filled with young, attractive—almost too attractive—women. He explained that these women were "dancers" from next door. That all the "dancers" were given free memberships to the gym.

I was young, impressionable, and almost broke at the time. But I became a member of that club that day. The latest equipment? Best trainers? Who cared? He sold me on the sights.

Rule 8: The Goal of the Free Orientation Is to Scare You

Don't be misled about what the free orientation you receive with your membership is for. It's not to get you acclimated to what the gym has to offer. It is not to teach you how to use the equipment. In fact, it's most often *completely* the opposite. You have already signed up. The gym has your money, for at least a year in most cases. You are now theirs. Yet it wants more. Much more.

That's right. The goal of the orientation at most gyms is not to educate you on how to work out, but rather to freak you out. Big time. To show you that you don't know squat. To make the gym out to be a scary, complicated place. To subtly convince you that you need help, lots of help. And that the trainer is just the person who can do it. For just $90 per hour. The more scared the person giving the orientation can make you, the more sessions he can ultimately sell you. Will it take twenty sessions to learn what you need to do? No way. You'll need at least a fifty-pack.

And while the trainer is hell-bent on freaking you out, he will also be prodding you for information. You may think it's just small talk, harmless banter, but it's not. He's conducting an investigation, gathering information on you. On what makes you tick. On what may motivate you.

He's looking for your "hot button."

What's a hot button? It's the incentive specific to you that he can exploit to sell you a few thousand dollars' worth of personal training.

Are you a woman getting married in six months? Holy cow, there's your hot button. And if he can't sell you sessions with that in your future, he needs to be fired on the spot. Uncovering an upcoming wedding during an orientation is like unearthing buried treasure. Jackpot!

"You're getting married? Congratulations! Wow, those are pictures that you will have for a lifetime. You really want to look great for those."

So the orientation is all about making you feel helpless and out of shape. Then the trainer is perfectly positioned to swoop in and save you.

Rule 9: Personal Trainers Are Promoted on the Basis of Sales, Not Certifications

I know, I know, That's not what the literature at your gym says. There are all sorts of "tiers"—different tiers for different trainers, supposedly based on education, experience, and number of certifications. The trainers who possess the most of all three criteria are supposed to be the "highest-level" trainer and therefore the most expensive.

Not at all.

It's simple economics. Gyms make lots and lots of money off of personal training. The more sessions they sell and the more expensive the sessions, the more money they make. If they have a trainer who is in demand, it behooves the gym to "promote" that person as fast as possible. The mere fact that the trainer has many clients gives off the impression that he or she must be really good at training, whereas in fact he or she may just be really good at selling. Quite often the quality of the trainer is inversely proportional to how expensive that person is.

Rule 10: If Your Trainer Looks as if He's on Steroids, He Probably Is

I've worked with many, many trainers who were taking steroids or who had taken them in the past. They were big, too big. Unnaturally large. A little too perfect. As your mother told you, if it looks too good to be true, it most often is. Don't be fooled. It never ceases to amaze me how few "real" people can tell when someone is on steroids.

There are now many different pharmaceuticals that can help you get bigger and more "ripped" with less effort in a short period of time. Thanks to the Internet, they have become much easier to get. Human growth hormone, testosterone, you name it, you can get it.

Trainers who take steroids drive me crazy. They are cheating, they are potentially damaging their bodies, and they have created a body that is a lie. They tell their clients that if they do their workouts they too can have a body like theirs, but they leave out the most important ingredient: Fitness is supposed to be about being as healthy as possible. Not as huge as possible.

Rule 11: If Your Gym Offers Overnight Locker Rentals, Rent a Locker

I can't emphasize enough how important this is. It can make the difference between your using the gym once every two weeks or five times *per* week.

Many gyms have both daily-use lockers that you can use for free and overnight lockers that you can rent by the month or year. Though it might seem like a frivolous expense, it is not. If you can afford to rent a locker, even if it seems a little expensive, do it. Doing so will increase the number of times you work out exponentially. You can stock it with everything you need: clothes, sneakers, deodorant, hairbrush, toothbrush, even postworkout bars and drinks. Whether you go to the gym or not depends on its convenience. The more convenient you make your gym experience, the more likely you are to go. In the end this smaller investment will make the bigger overall investment pay much bigger dividends. If you work, say good-bye to dragging a big bag to and fro each day. How great is that? You won't have to worry about forgetting your sneakers. You can use your own shampoo.

Many gyms that have lockers for rent also offer laundry service. It usually works like this: You are given a mesh bag with your locker number on it. You put your dirty clothes in the mesh bag and put the bag in the laundry. You then open your locker the next time you come to the gym and, voilà, there are your clothes, clean and ready to go. If you can swing it, do it. Having your own locker makes all the difference in the world.

2.

Sometimes It *Is* about the Bike: The Truth about Cardio, Stretching, and More

If you are going to BEAT THE GYM, you are going to have to "go hard and go home." Burn, baby, burn. If you really want to achieve the body of your dreams—or just be fit, for that matter—you have to burn calories through cardiovascular exercise. Here is one dictionary definition of cardiovascular exercise:

> **A system of physical conditioning designed to enhance circulatory and respiratory efficiency that involves vigorous sustained exercise.**

Vigorous. Sustained. Remember these two words. They are extremely important and two of the secrets to your long-term success. One of the major problems with fitness today is the myths and misconceptions about aerobic activity.

Sweat in the City

Karen had worked with dozens of trainers before coming to me, and she had tried all the fad diets. Though she had enjoyed modest successes from her efforts over the years, nothing had really worked. She wasn't doing it right. And cardio? She was walking several times a week with friends. Just walking.

She was a busy executive and mother with no time to waste. Her primary goal was to lose weight and tone up, just like most of you. And she wanted it done fast. Also like most of you.

Her secondary goal was to have the energy and stamina that her demanding job required. And relieve some stress in the process.

So we began running. Or should I say walk/jogging. Every other day. She could barely jog for a few minutes straight when we began, and she was a smoker. So we started slowly, running for a minute or two, then walking for a few minutes more, and repeating this pattern over and over. We did basic strength moves at the end. Soon the run intervals became longer and the walk intervals shorter. We varied the distances and varied the pace. We threw in intervals, and we threw in hills.

Over time, she smoked less. Her eating habits improved. We did a 5K race together, then a 10K. When we finished the 10K I turned to her and remarked that I thought she could do a marathon. Her husband, who was at the finish line at the time, said she could never do it.

We ran five marathons together, ran off an enormous amount of stress, and increased her energy level exponentially. She lost a significant amount of weight. She got rid of the bad smoking habit. And she got rid of the husband who didn't believe in her.

Rule 1: Do Not Use the "Fat-Burning" Programs on the Cardio Machines; They Will Keep You Fat

It's pretty darn simple, when it comes down to it: you get out what you put in. Work out hard, and you will burn a significant amount of calories. Go easy, and you won't. I want to pull out my hair when I read the books that tell you if you want to lose weight, you have to stay in your "fat-burning zone."

Fat-burning zone? Please.

I know, I know. You see posters illustrating the so-called fat-burning zone on the walls of your gym. They're on the displays of the cardio machines. For Pete's sake, they have "fat-burning" workouts programmed into the machines themselves. How could it be wrong?

Trainer Tip: You don't get more by doing less.

It's simply fuzzy math. Confusing, fuzzy math. Let me explain it for you.

When you work out at a lower intensity, say 60 percent of your maximum heart rate, your body burns primarily fat as fuel. Sounds great, right? As your cardio exercise increases in intensity, the body gradually shifts from burning fat to burning carbohydrate as fuel. So some misinformed fitness experts go on to tell you that one of the reasons you are not losing weight is that—get this—you are working out *too hard*.

That's right. Just go easier, and the pounds will drop off.

Have they lost their minds?

As with most outrageous diet and exercise claims, this one begins with some truth to it. It's true that our bodies burn more fat at lower intensities and more carbohydrate as we work harder. But—here's the kicker—what we're talking about here is *percentages.* And we're not taking into account total calories burned.

Confused? Don't be. It's simple. We burn a higher *percentage* of calories from fat at lower intensities. As you sit watching television, guess what? You are burning almost all your calories from fat. As we work out harder, however, we burn more total fat calories and more total calories overall. It's all about the totals. Here it is in simple mathematical terms.

> Workout 1, 30 minutes easy cardio: 250 total calories burned with 20 grams of fat; 72 percent of calories burned are from fat.

> Workout 2, 25 minutes intense cardio: 330 total calories burned with 25 grams of fat; 68 percent of calories burned are from fat.

So it is true. By working out easier, you burn a higher percentage of calories from fat. But by pushing the intensity you not only burn more fat calories, you burn more total calories as well. And when it comes to weight loss, it's all about burning more each day than you take in. Your caloric expenditure must exceed your caloric intake. This is known as a negative energy balance. We want to be negative when it comes to shedding unwanted pounds.

One more example I use to demonstrate this point. Have you ever watched a marathon—or any running race, for that matter? Who's heavier, the people at the front or the people at the back?

Sure, it's a flimsy analogy. But it makes the point. Don't kid yourself: when it comes to getting into shape, hard work is rewarded.

Rule 2: Traditional Heart Rate Zone Charts Are Wrong

If you thought the fat-burning zone was inaccurate, it pales in comparison to the recommended heart rate zones. The two are in fact connected. Heart rate zones are usually illustrated using color-coded charts, divided by age, that tell you what range you should try to stay within during your workout. There are several formulas that are used to compute these zones, with the most popular being the "age-graded heart rate formula." The formula is simple: subtract your age from 220 to determine your maximum heart rate. This is supposed to be the highest heart rate you can achieve during exercise.

Don't believe it.

Research indicates that a significant portion of the population, often said to be almost two-thirds, falls outside these zones. This means that a large number of you who are following the zones are in essence working out incorrectly. You are working out either too easy or too hard, and the chances are very good that it is the former. You are not working out at a high enough intensity.

You are ripping yourself off.

I have a client named Cooper: 37 years old, hedge fund guy, athletic. According to the age-based heart rate zones, his maximum heart rate should be:

220 – 37 [his age] = 183 beats per minute

I have measured his heart rate repeatedly during workouts. When he's really pushing hard, he can hit 210. *210.* I think he even has a few more beats left in him. During a recent comfortably hard run, he averaged 188 beats per minute.

That's five beats above the maximum his heart is supposed to be able to pump.

If he were to train in the so-called fat-burning zone, around 65 percent of his maximum heart rate, he would try to keep it around:

220 – 37 [age] = 183 [maximum heart rate] × 65% = 118

He'd be walking. Slowly.

Which leads right into the next rule:

Rule 3: Walking Is Not Exercise

Don't shoot the messenger just yet. Let me qualify this by stating that walking is a great activity if you:

1. Have a significant amount of weight to lose

2. Want to maintain basic cardiovascular health

3. Are deconditioned, elderly, injured, or just beginning an exercise program

But walking alone will not be enough to radically change your body. Or even maintain your weight in many cases. It goes back to simple math: the number of calories you expend by walking is just not enough to play a significant role in weight management, especially given today's American diet. We have taken so much of the activity out of our daily lives that walking as much as possible is the least we can do. But for the vast majority of you, it's not true exercise.

A Venti White Chocolate Crème Frappuccino Blended Beverage with whipped cream from Starbucks has . . . drumroll, please . . . *760 calories*. To *run* that off would take the average person more than an hour. Walking? You'd have to walk for a good three hours or so.

Rule 4: Get Your Heart Rate Up and Keep It Up

Remember the judge who gave his definition of pornography? He said he would know it when he saw it? Well, intensity during cardio is pretty much the same thing. How do you know when you're working out at an intensity that will bring about real results?

You'll know it when you feel it.

That's pretty much the rule when it comes to doing cardio. Push yourself. Burn away the calories. Create a negative daily caloric balance by expending more calories than you take in each and every day.

The Top Excuses Trainers Hear

I have heard it all when it comes to fitness-related excuses. Everything. From the obvious to the ridiculous to the downright baffling. Here are the top things trainers hear that keep people from getting into shape:

1. **I HAVE NO TIME.** Stop. Enough is enough. I don't care who you are or what you do, you have time. The average American watches something like three hours of television daily, yet the most common excuse for not working out is lack of time. A disconnect? I don't care who you are, you can get up thirty minutes earlier. Studies have consistently shown that getting in a workout first thing in the morning gives you more energy, not less.

   My best clients are the busiest. You need to make your workout a priority. Are you a busy mother who thinks she can't take time away from her children? Your kids will thank you for getting your workout in. Trust me. You will reduce your stress level and be a calmer, more patient mother as a result of your workout.

   Don't wait until you have a health issue to find the time to exercise. Do it now.

2. **I HAVE A SLOW METABOLISM.** Even if you do, which is most commonly self-diagnosed or diagnosed by someone with questionable credentials, so what? The weight gain attributable to this, even if true, is not a significant percentage. And most important? If you believe you have a slow metabolism, there is one surefire cure: eat less.

   As my crazy friend Chris likes to say, "It's not your metabolism, it's your fork."

   Having a slow metabolism means you don't need as many calories. Remember, it's about energy intake and energy expenditure. If you burn less, you need less, so you should consume less.

   This is also the very reason you should be focusing on strength training. Muscle is more metabolically active than fat. That means that the more lean muscle you have, the more calories you burn 24/7. Without doing anything. So you can actually speed up your metabolism, revving up your fat-burning engine, through exercise.

3. **I EAT REALLY WELL BUT STILL CAN'T LOSE WEIGHT.** Liar, liar, pants on fire. Once again, you need to get honest about what you eat. Snacks, drinks, handfuls of this and that, everything. Ever watch the show *Survivor*? The contestants are stuck in

remote locations for several weeks, with limited access to food, and the pounds fall off each and every one of them. It's a great illustration of how much we all consume and how every body type will lose weight when subjected to caloric restriction. Become cognizant of everything—and I mean everything—that passes your lips.

Over the years I have listened to hundreds and hundreds of people tell me what they "think" they eat. What I want to tell them is not to bother. I know what they eat. I'm looking at them.

4. I'VE BEEN BUSTING MY BUTT BUT STILL AM NOT SEEING RESULTS. Then you haven't been working out long enough, or at the right intensity, or with the right exercises. Or all three. It amazes me how many people think that they should see major changes after just a few weeks of working out. You didn't gain twenty pounds in a month, and you won't lose it in that amount of time, either. You may also be doing your cardio at the wrong intensity. Or your overall program design may be flawed. The bottom line is that if you are working out correctly and at the right intensity, you will absolutely see results. Follow the plans outlined in this book, and you won't need this excuse. Ever.

5. I DON'T WANT TO GET BULKY. Fear of the "B" word is one of the main reasons women avoid certain exercises and exercise routines and one of the primary reasons they don't achieve their best bodies. It drives me batty when I hear a woman fretting about getting "big." Being bulky is caused by excess fat, not by building "big" muscles. Not only are you deceiving yourself by avoiding certain exercises for fear of building too much muscle, you are keeping yourself from having the body you always wanted.

The bottom line is that you've got to get real. Stop kidding yourself. Let the excuses go. Not seeing the results you want? Then you need to change. Change not only what you are doing but, more important, what you are thinking when it comes to your workouts.

Debunking the Cardio Machines

Walk into the cardio area of most any gym today, and you can work up a sweat just trying to decide which piece of cardio equipment to use. Striders, stepmills, skiers, the StairMaster. Fitness companies are forever coming out with new and unique ways in which we can torture ourselves cardiovascularly.

Do you want to use your hands, or would you rather exercise with just your lower body like a cast member of *Riverdance*? The days of just the treadmill and StairMaster are long gone. If you can't find one type of cardio machine that you can tolerate a few times a week, you've got to get with the program. And, with so many choices available, many people inevitably want to know "Which is best?"

In fitness, when someone asks "Which is best?" what they really mean is "What can I do for the least amount of time and look absolutely fantastic as a result?" For cardio, this question translates into "Which piece of cardio equipment burns the most calories in the shortest amount of time?" The honest answer is threefold: it is whatever you do consistently, correctly, and at a significant intensity.

Rule 5: Consistency + Correct Use + Intensity = Cardio Success

1. **CONSISTENCY:** Nike got it half right with its famous slogan "Just do it." It needs to be expanded upon slightly to "Just do it consistently." Not once a month. Not every two weeks. Consistently.

2. **CORRECT USE:** This means using the machine with proper form. As Eric Clapton sang, no cheating. Don't jack the treadmill to an incline of 10 percent, then hold on to the display for dear life. For you StairMaster users and steppers, the same holds true. Do not put it on the highest level and then hold your body up on the handrails, performing what amounts to a triceps dip for an hour.

    Not only will using the machines improperly diminish your results, it can often lead to injury.

3. **AT A SIGNIFICANT INTENSITY:** As I stated earlier, you need to work out at a challenging level. This doesn't mean that you should be near death when

you are exercising. Let's put it this way: I see many people flipping through magazines while they ride the stationary bike or work out on the elliptical trainer. A good rule of thumb is that if you can read while you are doing cardio, you are not working out hard enough. Leave the magazines alone. Put on some music, jack up the intensity, get those endorphins flowing, and start transforming your body.

Rule 6: If You Can Read During Cardio, It Is Too Easy

While sweating is not a requirement to show that you are working out at a good intensity, many people who should be sweating during their cardio are not. *Many* people.

Not sweating may not show that you are taking it easy, but sweating certainly will indicate otherwise. When in doubt, sweat.

Now that you know the general principles of doing cardio, let's look at all the different choices available to you in most gyms. There are four tried-and-true machines that have been around for a while and will be around for many years to come.

The Treadmill

Or, as some like to refer to it, the "dreadmill." The treadmill is one of the best ways to burn the most calories. Why? Unlike on other machines, such as the elliptical trainer and the new treadclimbers, on the treadmill you have to completely support your body weight. With this significant benefit comes a cost, however: Some people cannot run due to the higher-impact forces involved. Their joints are not strong enough to handle the stress.

For those who cannot jog or run, the treadmill can also be used for walking. I know I just got through stating that walking is not exercise; well, if you must walk, the treadmill allows you to control both the speed and the incline. By manipulating these two variables, you can increase your calorie burn without causing undue stress on weaker joints.

The following are commonly found on treadmill displays:

Harder Treadmill —Good

1. Time

2. Distance

3. MPH (miles per hour)

4. Pace (per mile)

5. Heart rate

6. Incline

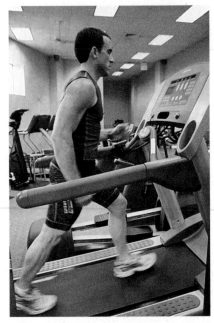

Most of the information displayed on the treadmill is self-explanantory. You want to go as far as possible as fast as possible, whether walking or running. The two ways to change the intensity of your treadmill routine are by increasing the speed and increasing the incline. Many treadmills are also compatible with heart-rate straps such as those made by Polar, so you can wear one and see your heart rate displayed on the screen.

Etiquette Tip: Never walk away from a treadmill while it is running.

This is really dangerous. As a trainer, I have seen dozens of people step unawares onto a treadmill that was running while the previous exerciser was getting a drink of water, running to the bathroom, or talking to someone across the gym floor. They have no idea the belt is moving, step onto it, and are immediately slammed onto their face and shot off into the wall behind them. It doesn't matter if you are running to the bathroom for thirty seconds; hit the pause button or turn the machine off altogether.

Trainer Tip: A 0.0 incline on most treadmills is slightly downhill. Set the incline to 1.0 to simulate a flat surface and burn more calories.

Rule 7: Running on a Treadmill Is Not the Same as Running Outside

Running on a treadmill is slightly easier than running outside for several reasons: you don't have to deal with changing terrain, wind resistance, and the ground moving underneath you.

TRAINER TIPS FOR GETTING THE MOST OUT OF YOUR TREADMILL WORKOUT

1. Set the incline to at least 1.0.
2. Do not hold on to the rails or display.
3. Do not read while working out.
4. Challenge yourself at different intensities.
5. Vary your workouts.

Trainer Tip: Do not hold dumbbells to make your workout more difficult.

Though I applaud the desire to work harder, this is one instance where it can be too much. Holding weights while walking or running on the treadmill can throw your natural stride off. Your body will be forced to compensate in a negative way, which can lead to injury. Stick to increasing the speed and/or the incline to make your cardio sessions more challenging.

Etiquette Tip: Ask before changing the channel on a shared TV.

Many gyms have rows of cardio machines with numerous television monitors in front of them. You plug your headphones into a box on your machine and then tune in to the channel of the TV you want to watch during your workout. Usually this is a monitor relatively close to the machine you

Treadmill—Bad

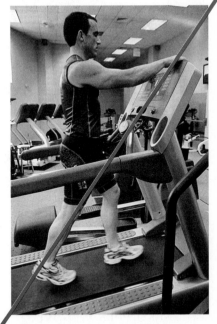

No draping your body over the display or holding on while you walk. If you have to hold on, it's too fast, too steep, or both.

will be using. If the channel on the TV in front of your treadmill is set to the Food Channel and you'd like to watch *Law & Order*, you have to check to make sure no one is watching how to make a raspberry sorbet. Here is the proper protocol: Stand under the TV and face the cardio equipment. Point up at the monitor and ask if anyone minds if you can change the channel. Scan the room while waiting for a response. If anyone says yes, he or she is watching. Then move to another machine. If no objection is made, feel free to turn on your show.

Rule 8: Running Does Not Cause Osteoarthritis

Shocked to hear this? Most people are. There now exists definitive empirical evidence in the form of longitudinal studies that show that runners have a *lower* incidence of osteoarthritis than their nonrunning counterparts. One of the main reasons for this is that runners weigh significantly less than nonrunners. You know what is really tough on the joints? Carrying twenty, thirty, fifty excess pounds around twenty-four hours a day, seven days a week.

Etiquette Tip: Don't forget to wipe.

Wipe down your cardio machine after you use it. You might think that this tip doesn't need mentioning, but it most certainly does. Cardio machines are constantly left covered in sweat by inconsiderate gymgoers. It's just gross. When you are finished with your workout, just take your workout towel or a few paper towels and wipe away all the sweat. Some gyms have spray bottles of products that you can use to clean the equipment.

My sweat rate is so high that not only is my treadmill completely coated with sweat, I also hit the treadmills on either side and the one behind me as well. I'm pretty much like Shamu at SeaWorld; there is a "splash zone" all around me. Suffice it to say that people who know me avoid being anywhere near me during my cardio sessions. But I wipe up every single drop of sweat I create. It just takes a while.

The Stationary Bike

For those who either can't or don't want to use the treadmill, the stationary bike is a great alternative. Your body is supported, and there is much less impact on the joints. Just as with the treadmill, you want to vary your workouts on the bike.

Some days just ride easy, other days do short intervals and long tempos, and throw a hill workout in every now and again as well.

There are two basic types of bikes in the gym; upright and recumbent. The upright bike has you more vertical, while the recumbent bike positions your body more horizontally. The benefit of the recumbent bike is that it supports your back and can be a little more comfortable than an upright. The downside is that you have to work harder to get your heart rate up on the recumbent bike. So if your goal is to burn the maximum number of calories, choose the upright bike.

Trainer Tip: To really tone those glutes, get "out of the saddle."

For women who really want to tone their lower bodies, especially their glutes, the stationary bike is a phenomenal tool. One great workout to target the tush is hills. Alternate between seated hills and hills "out of the saddle," meaning you are standing and really pushing down on the pedals.

DECODING THE BIKE DISPLAY

The following are commonly found on stationary bike displays:

1. Time
2. Distance
3. Speed
4. Heart rate
5. RPMs
6. Level
7. Watts

The first four are straightforward: how long you have been working out, how far you have traveled, how fast you are going, and how high your heart rate is. To get your heart rate, you need to be either holding the sensors found on the handles of many stationary bikes or wearing a heart-rate monitor strap that is compatible with the machine.

RPMs, which stands for "revolutions per minute," tells you how many times

Footwear

Fitness is full of contradictory information. That's one of the reasons there is so much confusion involved with getting into shape. What are you to believe? Well, just when you think the shoe manufacturers have running shoes figured out, they go and pull a 180 on the whole concept of footwear. Nike and the top shoe manufacturers have been designing shoes to support our arches, control our pronation or supination, absorb shock, provide stability.

Now the latest research is saying that shoes may be doing *too much;* they could potentially be the *cause* of many running-related injuries.

Great. More confusion, right?

Running Shoes

The newest running shoes on the market look like slippers and provide little to no support. The new theory being promoted is that we need to allow our feet to feel the ground, make natural biomechanical adjustments, and strengthen themselves over time. Shoes like the Vibram Five Fingers are now flying off the shelves. I have several pairs and love them. I use them for short distances. You can't go out and run six miles in these shoes right away. I use Asics for my longer runs and the Vibrams for shorter workouts.

What shoes are right for you? And where should you buy them? Go to a running specialty store that is staffed by runners. They will ask you a handful of questions, let you try on several pairs of shoes, examine the wear pattern on your old shoes, and possibly even put you on a treadmill and observe your running form or "gait."

The best shoe is the one that fits you best. There is no one perfect shoe for everybody. The best shoe for you depends on a variety of factors, including your goals, weight, biomechanics, arch type, surface you'll be exercising on, amount you'll be exercising, and more. Get fitted at a store that specializes in running shoes.

Spin Shoes

One of the things about spin class that scares people away is the shoes. They see the "hard-core" spinners clomping around in their special bike shoes with the cleats on the bottom and think the class is too advanced for them. It isn't, trust me.

Do you need spin shoes? The short answer is no. Most spin bikes have double-sided pedals: on one side there is a clip for the spin shoes, on the other side is a cage for you to slide your sneakers into. Both work. You can burn calories and have a great time wearing either type of shoe.

If you decide you like spinning and start to do it several times a week, you may want to try out some spin shoes. There is a different "feel" to them, and you can pedal more efficiently when you are secured to the pedal. Go to your local bike shop and tell the people there that you want shoes for spin class. You don't have to break the bank, either. Let's be honest: you're pedaling on a bike that's not going anywhere.

Cross-Training Shoes

If you are taking classes like boot camp, circuit training, and step-based workouts, you may want to leave the running shoes at home. These classes require a bit more cushioning and lateral support, something that your lighter-weight running shoe may not provide. Yes, there are different shoes for different applications. I tried wearing my running shoes in a cardio kickboxing class recently and found them to be too flimsy and lightweight for the workout. Tell your qualified shoe salesperson specifically what you will be doing in the shoes and have him recommend footwear appropriate for the demands of the workout.

Shower Shoes

You can in fact catch certain "things" by walking around the gym's locker rooms, shower, steam rooms, and saunas barefoot. Plantar warts, for one. It's a good idea to get into the habit of wearing sandals, inexpensive rubber ones, while in the locker rooms. It can save you a not-so-fun trip to the podiatrist in the future.

the pedal crank makes one complete circle. Another term for RPMs is "cadence." When the resistance is low, your RPMs will be higher. When the resistance is high, as when you are climbing a hill, your RPMs will drop.

"Level" is simply a benchmark of resistance. The higher the level, the greater the intensity. If you were to do a workout that incorporated hills, you would raise and lower the level to simulate riding up and down inclines. The longer you can stay at a specific level and the easier that level feels, the stronger you are becoming. Also, the lower your heart rate is at any given level, the fitter you are. If during one workout your average heart rate is 160 at level 6 and several weeks later it is 150, this shows that your fitness level has increased; your heart has to do less work against the same workload.

"Watts" is a measurement of energy. Think of a lightbulb. The greater the number of watts, the more energy it puts out. Cyclists are now training more and more by wattage. The more watts you can sustain for any given period of time, the stronger you are. The riders in the Tour de France average insanely high wattages for their rides. You can use watts to gauge the intensity of your workouts as well as design your workouts. You may warm up by averaging 150 watts, then do intervals of keeping the watts above 200, then cool down back at 150 watts.

You can also use average watts to see improvements in your fitness. If you average 175 watts during one bike workout and then 182 watts for the same workout a few weeks later, this shows improvement.

Rule 9: When You Can Keep Your RPMs at a Higher Number for a Longer Time at a Particular Level, You Are Getting Stronger

Once again, "Level" on the bike refers to the amount of tension you will be pedaling against. The higher the level, the greater the resistance. The greater the resistance, the harder the workout. When you can keep pedaling at higher RPMs at the same level, that is another sign you are getting fitter.

Trainer Tip: Take advantage of coached cardio workouts.

Thanks to MP3 players, you can now have a "cardio coach" guide your workout through your personal music player. These workouts, which you can order on CDs or download from the Internet, have a person coaching you while you train on the elliptical trainer, treadmill, stationary bike, whatever. Set over a musical sound track, the coach will give you cues on intensity, speed, resistance, intervals, hills, visualization, and more to help you get the most out of your cardio session. Coached workouts are great because they provide structure and intensity to your workouts that you most likely wouldn't achieve on your own. I have a few of my own that you can download for free on www.teamholland.com. Another great site for these audio workouts is www.cardiocoach.com.

Fit Myth: The bike will make your legs bulky.

Not true. The bike is an incredible way to help shape and tone your lower body, giving you the best legs you are genetically capable of having.

The StairMaster

It has been in the gym for years, the tried-and-true old StairMaster. StairMaster is a brand name and the popular original stair workout; numerous steppers and treadclimbers have followed. I personally still love the original. It is extremely effective, and it's not easy when done correctly. The only problem is it's rarely ever used the way it was designed.

I received my undergraduate degree from Boston College and have vivid memories of rows of people sweating away on the StairMasters in our gym, especially in the weeks before spring break. They were working out feverishly in a desperate attempt to lose a few pounds before they had to squeeze into a bathing suit. Almost all of them had the StairMaster cranked up to the highest level. Not strong enough to sustain the pace with their legs alone, they all held on to the handrails with their arms locked out, tiptoeing on the pedals. They were getting almost nothing out of the exercise.

StairMaster—Bad

Trainer Tip: Here's how to get the most out of the StairMaster.

Correct form is so rarely used on the StairMaster. This is amazing to me, given how long this machine has been around. The proper and effective technique for using it is to use the full range of the pedal stroke: pushing it all the way down until it almost touches the floor, then bringing it all the way up until it almost touches the top of the pedal stroke. Doing this full motion requires activating all the leg muscles, especially the glutes. The improper manner in which the majority of people work out on the StairMaster changes it into a calf and triceps exercise, with a minimal caloric expenditure.

If you want to burn a significant number of calories while toning your entire lower body, get on the StairMaster and use it correctly. It's an awesome piece of cardio equipment.

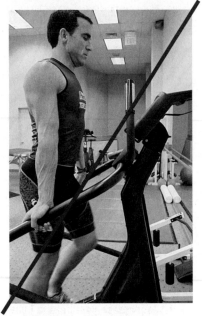

Are you working your triceps or your legs? Let go of the handles.

Fit Myth: The StairMaster makes your butt big.

Nope. A big butt is the direct result of eating too much and exercising too little.

The Elliptical Trainer

Incredibly enough, the elliptical trainer first entered the market in the 1990s. It is amazing to me that it took that long to invent this machine. The elliptical trainer is essentially for those who want a cardio workout with significantly less stress on their joints than they would get on a treadmill. This reduced strain is due to the oval or elliptical motion, which provides support to the body. Elliptical trainers come with or without arm attachments. Certain models allow you to adjust the incline, resistance, and stride length.

There is debate on the caloric expenditure of the elliptical trainer versus the treadmill. Some studies indicate that when one is using an elliptical trainer with the arm attachments, the caloric expenditure is the same as on a treadmill, while the perceived exertion is lower. In other words, you get the same results on the elliptical trainer while feeling as though you are doing less.

Personally, I'm not sold on that theory. I've said it before: when it comes to fitness, you don't get more by doing less. It's just not the way the world works.

I think the invention of the elliptical trainer was a great thing. It allows a huge group of people who couldn't or wouldn't do cardio before the opportunity to get healthy. Given that the elliptical trainer is relatively new when it comes to exercise equipment, I'm not convinced that there is enough data on the caloric expenditure yet. It all comes down to the formulas the manufacturers program into the equipment. I think more research needs to be done before they can accurately dial them in.

Trainer Tip: Increase your calorie burn when using an elliptical trainer by using the arm attachments.

To increase your calorie burn when using the elliptical trainer, use the arm attachments. The more body parts that are moving, the more weight you will lose.

More Cardio Machines

The four machines mentioned above are the mainstays in most gyms. In addition to them are the following machines that you can also work up a sweat on.

The "Erg" Rowing Machine

I have to admit, I'm not an erg guy. Never have been. I used one a couple of times back when I was eighteen during my first job at the local YMCA. I found it to be really difficult and have not been on it since. My editor, on the other hand, loves this mode of cardiovascular torture. So do many others, and for good reason: it provides a phenomenal cardiovascular workout involving the entire body. We just ordered another for my club to keep up with the demand.

It has a flywheel that you can adjust to simulate the feel of rowing on the water. You sit on it, put your feet into straps, and hold on to a handle attached to a chain. In one smooth motion you pull the handle while pushing away from the flywheel with your lower body. It takes coordination and practice to get it just right. Do not overdo your first few sessions on the erg. Do five minutes or so at an easy intensity.

Fit Myth: The erg is all about the upper body.

Most nonrowers think the erg is all about the upper body. This is not true. Rowing is a much more complex movement. The erg actually provides a full-body workout that involves the legs much more than people realize. The core as well. It requires a smooth transfer from the lower body, through the core, and then to the upper body.

Proper form is crucial, as bad technique can injure the lower back.

The standard measurement on the erg is known as the "split," the amount of time required to travel five hundred meters at the current pace.

The display on the erg often shows such data such as stroke count, total strokes, time elapsed, resistance, and calories burned.

TIPS ON USING THE ERG

1. Be sure to strap your feet securely into the footrests.
2. Do not round your back while rowing. Sit up straight with good posture and bend slightly from the waist.
3. Focus on pushing with your legs.
4. Keep the resistance low if you are using it for the first time.
5. Switch your grip occasionally. Row sometimes with your palms up, other times with your palms down.
6. Pull the handle until it is almost touching your stomach and your elbows pass behind your body.

The NordicTrack

It's the old wooden cross-country skiing machine. Yes, they can still be found in some gyms, including mine. There is always one, sometimes two, members who are fanatical about their NordicTrack. It's all they use, and if you get rid of it, they will quit the gym.

It takes a bit of coordination, however, to get the legs working in synchronization with your arms. You slide wooden skis from front to back while pulling on cables that are your "poles." It's actually a great workout if you can do it. It's easy on the joints, yet you can really get your heart rate up if your push the intensity. Cross-country skiing is one of the highest-calorie-burning activities there is. If your gym has one, try it out. You just may have to fight the die-hard guy who thinks it's his and only his.

Trainer Tip: If you want to use the NordicTrack and have a hard time getting the rhythm, don't try to do it all at once. Start with just the legs for thirty seconds or so, then add the arms.

The Gauntlet

One of my absolute favorite cardio machines. You know the one: The huge black behemoth usually tucked away in a dark, hot corner of the gym. It's the moving stairs, the ones that just keep coming and coming. Unlike the StairMaster and steppers, where you push down on pedals, the Gauntlet has stairs that actually rotate underneath you. It's a fantastic workout. It's very difficult to cheat on, it burns a heap of calories, and it is also a "functional" type of exercise.

Gauntlet—Bad

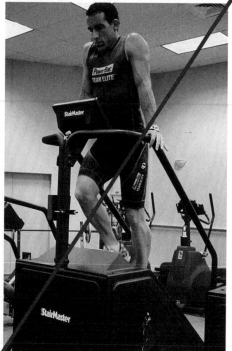

Once again, lose the arms.

Gauntlet—Good

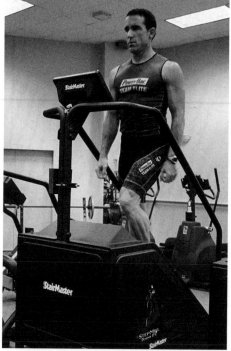

Pump your arms in a natural walking motion. You'll burn a heck of a lot more calories.

FUNCTIONAL EXERCISES: These are exercises that closely resemble movements involved in everyday activities, for example, squats and lunges. Doing such exercises makes the activities of daily living easier. They also help prevent injuries by increasing coordination and balance.

The only real way to cheat on the Gauntlet is to hang on to the siderails. But, unlike with the StairMaster or steppers, even if you do hold on, you still have to work hard to keep climbing up the moving stairs. To maximize your results on the Gauntlet, hold the rails lightly with just your fingertips, just to keep your balance. If you are particularly strong and coordinated, you can get even greater results by not holding on at all. Pump your arms at your sides in a natural motion, just as if you were climbing stairs in a building.

Trainer Tip: Want to make the Gauntlet even harder? Wear a weight vest while using it.

Upper-Body Ergometer

Most often found in rehabilitation facilities, upper-body ergometers are finding their way into more and more gyms as weekend warriors continue to injure themselves in greater numbers and the older population is using gyms more as well. These are cardio machines that involve only your arms. They are therefore great for people who are rehabbing a lower-body injury or those too frail to work out on traditional cardio machines. You sit on them and spin cranks with your arms, essentially "pedaling" with your upper body. There is no lower-body involvement at all. It is one of the few machines on which you can increase your heart rate and burn calories without using your legs. If you ever have a knee or hip injury and need to get your cardio in, the upper-body ergometer will be your best friend.

Etiquette Tip: Don't hog the equipment.

Some gyms have specific rules posted, such as "30-Minute Limit," especially during peak usage hours. You need to follow the rules. At extremely crowded gyms there may even be sign-up sheets for the cardio equipment. If your gym does not have specific rules posted, you should still be considerate and adhere to a thirty-minute rule if people are waiting.

And if you are waiting to get on a piece of cardio, please do not hover around and stare at the person who is currently using it. It creeps that person out and ruins his or her workout. You can politely ask the person how much time he or she has left and then ask to have it next if no sign-up procedure is in place.

1. Talking on a cell phone
2. Singing out loud
3. Making any unusual intermittent sound such as grunting
4. Staying on longer than the posted time limit
5. Not wiping off your sweat
6. Having bad body odor or exercising in stinky workout clothes
7. Passing gas

Rule 10: One Pound Equals 3,500 Calories

It's pretty simple: if your goal is to lose weight, then the more weight you want to lose, the more cardio you need to do. Remember that it all comes down to simple math. If you take one thing away from this book, it will be that *a pound equals 3,500 calories*. It never ceases to amaze me how few people know this fact. Whenever I am addressing a large group of people, as during a lecture or when I am leading my annual Nantucket Beach Fitness Camp, I always pose this question. Rarely do more than five out of a hundred people get it right.

So to lose a pound, you need a deficit of 3,500 calories. That's way more than people think. Let's put it this way: the general rule of thumb is that you burn roughly 100 calories for every mile you run. So if you run a ten-minute mile, you will burn around 600 calories in an hour.

To lose one pound, then, you would have to run for about *six hours.* The average marathon time is around four hours and forty minutes for women and around four hours for men. So if you were to run a marathon, you might lose one pound.

One pound.

Remember that exercise intensity changes the number of calories you burn: the harder and faster you go, the more calories you burn.

Rule 11: You Do Not Burn the Same Number of Calories Walking As You Do Running

You burn roughly half the number of calories walking a mile as you do running the same distance.

In case you need a guideline on how much cardio to do each week, I have come up with an extremely simple formula. For every pound you weigh, you need to do a minute of cardio. Super simple. So if you weigh 150 pounds, I want you to do 150 minutes of cardio per week. You can choose to split it up whatever way you wish: You can do five days of cardio for thirty minutes each session, two sessions each lasting one hour plus one thirty-minute session, and so on. You can even do one session of two and a half hours if you leave it to the last minute.

This formula works on several important levels:

1. It's simple.

2. It factors in your weight. The heavier you are, the more cardio you should be doing to get rid of the excess pounds.

3. It allows you the freedom to break up the workouts any way that works for you. I can't stress how important this point is. If you feel like doing a long session one day, great. If you can get in only fifteen minutes in on another, that works too. Want to do two twenty-minute sessions in one day, one in the morning, one after work? No problem. But you must have a plan. In a seven-day cycle you must get the allotted number of minutes in.

4. Over time you are rewarded by having to do less. The more consistent you are, the more weight you will lose. The more weight you lose, the less time you have to spend doing cardio. It's a huge win-win. And, if you are already starting out at a light weight, you might have to do only 120 minutes of cardio per week and can spend more time on strength training.

To Stretch or Not to Stretch:
That Is the Question

Should you stretch? This is yet another topic in fitness where you will find strong arguments supporting both sides of the issue. It would make a phenomenal topic for a debate class. Much of the confusion has been caused by a small group of studies, which really don't apply to the majority of us who are trying to be fit and injury-free. The question needs to be rephrased to be not "*Should* we stretch?" but "*When, what,* and *how* should we stretch?"

The old-school method of stretching was the "static" method: standing on one leg, grabbing a toe, and pulling a heel toward your butt to stretch the front of your thigh. You then threw a heel up onto a chair or something similar and leaned into it to stretch your hamstrings, then pushed against a wall to loosen up the calves. There was no real thought involved. Why did we do it? Because we had done it that way in gym class and in sports and because we saw other people do it before exercise. Monkey see, monkey do.

Yes, we still need to stretch, but not necessarily *when* and *why* we originally thought.

Stretching before exercise? Not like that. You need to replace the term "stretch" with "warm-up" when it comes to preexercise stretching. Recent studies have shown that static stretching before exercise not only doesn't necessarily help, it may even cause injury. I'm not completely sold on the injury-causing part, but I do believe the "warm-up" theory.

You need to warm up your body before exercise, prime it for what is to come. This is achieved not by stretching the muscles in a static fashion but rather through a "dynamic warm-up." This is basically a short amount of cardio done before the real workout session. So, if you are doing a weight workout, you want to precede it with a low-level bout of cardio, such as riding a stationary bike or walking for three to five minutes. This dynamic warm up serves several functions, the most important being increasing blood flow to the muscles you are about to work and elevating your core temperature.

The same thing holds true for your cardio sessions. You should always begin with an easy warm-up of three minutes or longer at a low speed and intensity. Like a car that has been sitting in a cold garage overnight, you need to warm up before you open up and fire on all cylinders.

After this dynamic warm-up you can then stop and stretch quickly, performing the basic static stretches of the major muscle groups. Studies indicate that holding these stretches for just fifteen seconds or so is all you should do. But, again, you want to warm up the muscles with low-level full-body movement before doing these stretches.

After your workout? That's different. Your muscles are now warmed and pumped full of blood. You hopefully have a good sweat going, and your core temperature is up. Now you can spend a few minutes stretching the major muscle groups. Whereas you want to hold the stretches for ten to twenty seconds or so before your workout, spend thirty to sixty seconds on each muscle after exercise.

The stretching debate will rage on. That's fine with me. All I know is two things:

1. Repetitive motions cause muscles to shorten and become tight over time.

2. As we age, we lose flexibility and joint range of motion.

The more I run, the tighter I get. I know I feel better and run better when I work on my flexibility. Here is what I recommend you do when it comes to stretching before your strength and cardio workouts:

1. At least three minutes of a cardiovascular exercise done at a very low level of intensity

2. A quick stretch of the major muscles, holding each for fifteen seconds or so

3. Five to ten minutes of stretching postexercise, now holding each stretch for thirty to sixty seconds

Here's an easy way to mix up your cardio session that will benefit you physically as well as mentally. It doesn't matter if you are on a treadmill, an elliptical trainer, a stationary bike, whatever. While you are watching television, go at an easy, steady pace, about a 6 on a scale of 1 to 10, with 10 being really hard. Whenever there are commercials, increase your speed or the resistance up to an 8 or 9 on the same intensity scale, and keep it there during the entire break. When the show resumes, drop back down to the easy pace to recover. Repeat this for the entire workout. Think about it: if you watch your favorite thirty-minute show, this is a perfect way to get in a quality workout that includes a warm-up, several hard intervals, and a cooldown.

Rule 12: Mix Up Your Cardio. Often

We gravitate to doing what we like and what we are good at. This is one of the primary reasons we ultimately plateau and stop seeing results. Your body is an extremely intelligent machine and adapts quickly to the stressors placed on it. Not only do you need to vary the workouts you do on your favorite piece of cardio equipment, you also need to get off that machine occasionally and try something new. Here are some suggestions for how you can shake up your cardio routine:

If You Like . . .

- The bike, you should check out the treadmill. Biking works primarily the quadriceps, while the treadmill hits the hamstrings; thus these two exercises will keep these muscles in balance.

- The elliptical, you should check out the StairMaster or another kind of stepper. You will probably like the slightly similar yet different muscle activation.

- The treadmill, you should check out the stationary bike. Again, these two exercises work opposing muscle groups that, when out of balance, can lead to injury.

- The stepper, you should check out the stationary bike. Why? Why not? Mix it up.

Rule 13: Circuit Workouts Are Not Always the Answer

Mixing strength training with cardio is one of the best ways to maximize your workouts, but circuit workouts are not always the way to go. Sometimes we need (or want) to just lift weights. On other days straight cardio workouts are called for. It's kind of like peanut butter and chocolate for me. I love them both. But some days I want one or the other, while other days I want them together, as in Reese's Peanut Butter Cups. It's the same for cardio and strength training. Separate. Together. Both are good. Mix them up.

Four Great Workouts for Any Cardio Machine

Variation is one of the major keys to success when it come to getting in shape. Many people do the same exact workout day in and day out, then wonder why their bodies stop changing. You must constantly "confuse" your body, thus forcing it to adapt. The changes can be simple.

Treadmill, elliptical, stationary bike, it doesn't matter. You can take these four essential formats and work them into your program to stay mentally stimulated and keep your results coming.

1. **ENDURANCE:** Steady-state. Crank up the iPod, pick an easy pace, and go long. This is probably the workout you already do.

2. **HILLS:** After a warm-up, do a series of hills with a recovery after each one. Perform a short cooldown after the hills as well.

3. **INTERVALS:** After a warm-up, perform a series of short, fast intervals with a recovery after each one.

4. **TEMPO:** After a warm-up, do a longer, "comfortably hard" interval anywhere from five to thirty minutes in length. Do a short cooldown afterward.

Trainer Tip: Stretch in between sets.

Most of us hate to stretch, especially at the end of a workout. You just want the workout to be over; the last thing you want to do is spend another ten minutes or so stretching. Though you should still stretch out at the end of your exercise sessions, you can also occasionally stretch within a workout itself. What I like to do during some strength workouts is stretch between each set. You want to take thirty seconds or so rest between each set anyway, right? So why not kill two birds with one stone and spend that time stretching the muscle you just worked? For example, you would do one set in the extension machine, then get out and pull up on a foot, stretching each quadriceps for fifteen to thirty seconds. Get back into the leg extension machine, do another set, then get out and stretch again. By stretching the muscle you just worked after each set, you will improve your flexibility as well as maximize your time in the gym.

There are four major muscle groups in the lower leg that benefit from static stretching. Again, do these stretches between sets to maximize your workout time.

Quad Stretch

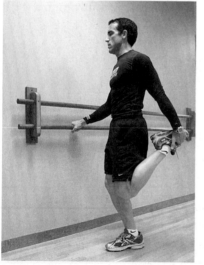

Stand upright and hold the toes of one foot as you gently pull your heel towards your butt. Keep your knees side by side; do not pull the leg back behind you or lean forward. You can bend your supporting leg slightly and push your hips forward. You should feel a gentle stretch in the front of your raised thigh.

Hamstring Stretch

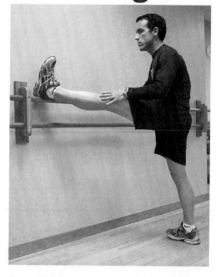

Place the heel of one leg on a sturdy raised object such as a bench or chair. Keeping this leg straight, press the heel down gently as you slowly lean forward with your upper body. You should feel a gentle stretch in the back of your thigh.

Warm-ups

Remember that static stretching before workouts is no longer the thing to do. We want to move, get the blood flowing, and warm up the muscles through low-level aerobic activity. Here are a few of my favorite ways to warm up a client:

1. Jumping jacks

2. Jumping rope

3. Running up stairs (slowly)

4. Doing walking lunges

Glute Stretch

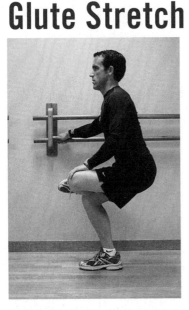

Holding on to an object such as a chair or bench for support, cross one ankle above your knee and slowly sit back as if you were lowering yourself down into a seated position. Stop when you feel a gentle stretch in the glute (butt muscle) of the leg that is raised and hold.

Calf Stretch

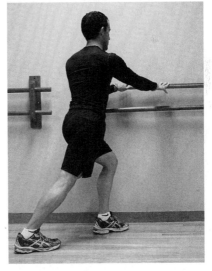

Stand with a staggered stance in front of an object such as a tree or a wall. Place your hands on the object for support and straighten your back leg. Gently press the heel of your back leg down into the ground while bending your front knee slowly forward. You should feel a gentle stretch in the back of your lower leg.

Rule 14: No One Ever Got Skinny from Doing Yoga or Pilates

Yoga and Pilates do have enormous benefits when it comes to overall health and well-being. I recommend them highly for building a specific type of strength, for increasing flexibility, and for creating body awareness.

It's simple science: A calorie is heat. Heat is energy. To lose weight, you need to increase your energy expenditure. And since a pound equals 3,500 calories, you need to significantly increase this expenditure in order to lose weight. Studies show that neither yoga nor Pilates raises your heart rate enough to burn this amount of calories. That's a fact. Don't shoot the messenger.

So what about the skinny women who take those classes?

1. They walked in the door that way.

2. They eat less than most other people do.

3.

Machines Are Your Friends and Dumbbells Will Make You Smart: The Surprisingly Not-Scary Facts About Strength Training

L ook around a gym; the view can be daunting. There are so many different machines, so many different pieces of equipment, and so many different ways to use them all. I understand your trepidation. I know how overwhelming it can be. I too was a beginner once. This fear is one of the main reasons people do the same workouts with the same machines over and over again. They do what they know (or think they know) and what they are good at. You are not alone.

But as you begin to BEAT THE GYM, you will start to look at the gym floor in a whole new light. You will see possibilities rather than confusion, opportunity rather than obstacles. Machines that frightened you in the past will get you excited—because you will know how to use them and how they can transform your body.

As a trainer I have two main goals with clients: to educate them and to empower them. This book will educate you on what you should do and how you should do it. You will then be empowered and able to walk into any gym at any time and use any piece of equipment. You can do it!

When you look around your gym, you probably see the following. First, an area with big, hulking strength machines: the leg press machine, the shoulder press machine, and so on. People are moving slowly from one station to the next, adjusting the machines, pushing and pulling, grunting and groaning. The machines are generally less frightening for most people than the free weights; you can watch others to see what to do. The machines often have a sign on them to help guide you through the movements. There's usually only one way to use them. But there is still confusion when it comes to the machines. This book will make this relatively safe area completely comfortable for you.

Next comes the free-weight area. This is much scarier for most people. There are more men in this part of the gym. Often big men. They are often letting out random yells while sweating all over the place. Weights are being thrown around. It's noisy. Sometimes smelly. Who wouldn't be intimidated by a place like this?

I love taking a woman who is afraid of exercising in this area and transforming her into "one of the guys." Someone who feels totally comfortable doing squats in the Smith machine and bench-pressing all on her own. Strong and confident. More capable than the majority of the men. *Beat the Gym* will help you become this person.

Then there is the stretching and abdominals area. People scattered across the rubber mats, pounding out push-ups, cranking out crunches on brightly colored balls, contorting their bodies to stretch overly tight muscles. While this area is much less frightening, it too is in need of major clarification. Some people perform lots of bad exercises and movements here. Others waste lots of time on those mats. *Beat the Gym* will ensure that you are not one of those people.

So read on. I will be your personal trainer, helping you to navigate through all these areas. I will help you become a seasoned pro, taking away the fear and uncertainty and transforming you into someone other people will approach for exercise advice.

The Secrets of Strength Training

Strength training: it's what I love, what I'm passionate about, and, if I say so myself, what I'm really good at. I love the tight feeling I get after a good full-body workout. I love seeing the changes I can make in my body by pushing and pulling weights around. I have studied those who are successful at it and emulated them.

What blows me away is that the vast majority of people lifting weights in the gym are doing it wrong. Really wrong. Most likely you are one of them. The time has come for you to stop wasting your time and to start getting results. Especially those of you who are going to the gym several times a week or more yet are still not seeing any real change. Enough is enough. I can help.

I'm going to break down the strength training area of the gym for you so that you can enjoy your workouts while getting the most out of every one of them. First, I'll break down the machines, then I'll show you free weights with dumbbells and barbells, followed by body-weight exercises. I'll go on to simplify strength training with cables, and we'll finish up with how to train your core. There will be pictures of the exercises so that you can see exactly what you'll be doing and the proper way to execute each movement. Your workouts will never be the same.

Lifting Lingo: Periodization

For athletes, "periodization" means the cycling of intensity and volume to maximize performance.

What does this mean for you? Think of it as simply that you need to mix up your routine. Constantly. Periodization is crucial both to getting results and to staying injury-free.

Selectorized Machines

These machines have weight stacks and a pin. You put the pin into the plate corresponding to the weight you want to lift, and off you go.

Machine Back Row

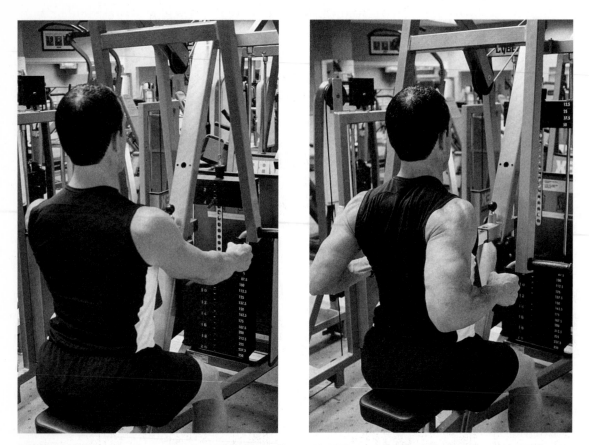

Sitting with perfect posture, pull the handles toward you, initiating the movement from your back. Keep your chest out and press your shoulder blades together. Hold for 1 second, then slowly return to the starting position.

Machine Shoulder Press

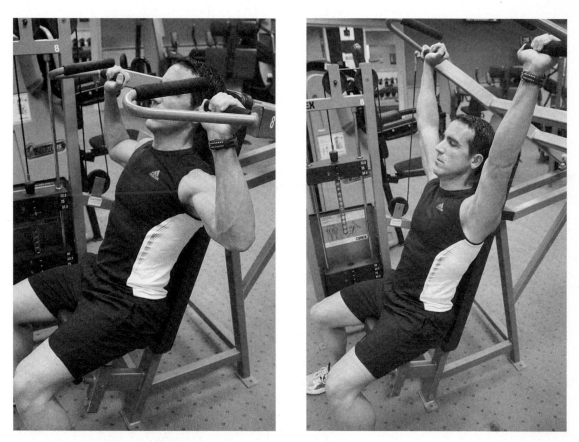

Press the handles up until your arms are fully extended, hold for 1 second, then slowly return to the starting position.

Machine Lateral Raise

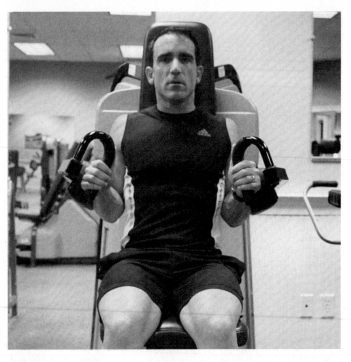

Raise the handles until your arms are in line with your shoulders, hold for 1 second, then slowly return to the starting position.

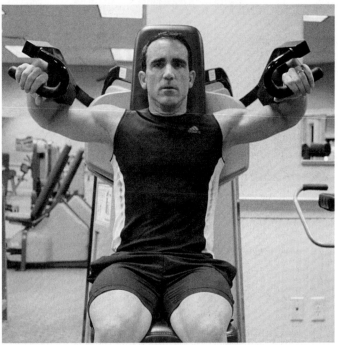

Machine Prone Leg Curl

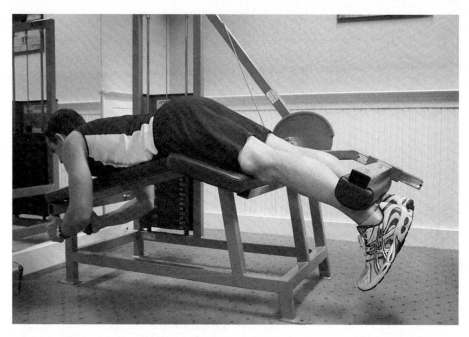

With the pad resting just above your ankles, curl the bar toward your butt, hold for 1 second, then slowly return to the starting position.

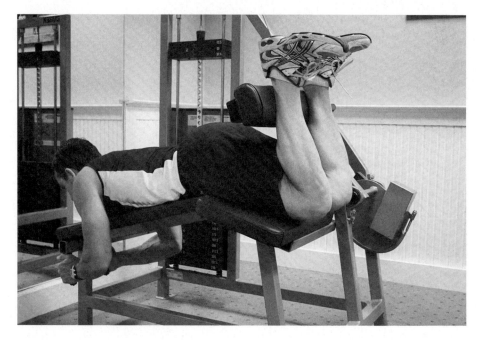

Single-Leg Machine Prone Leg Curl

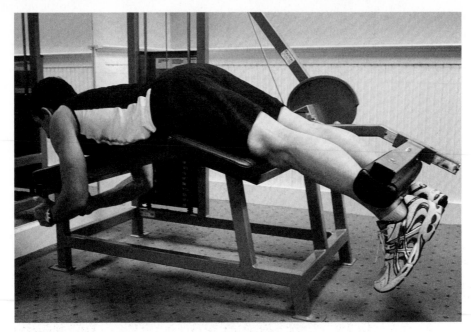

The same exercise, one leg at a time.

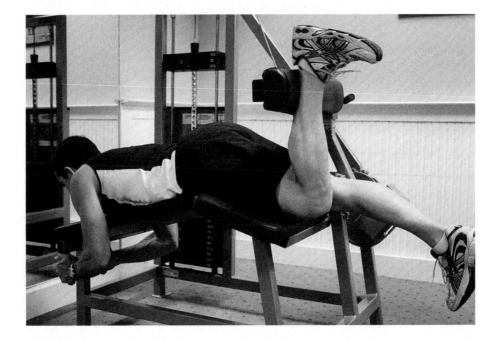

Machine Leg Extension

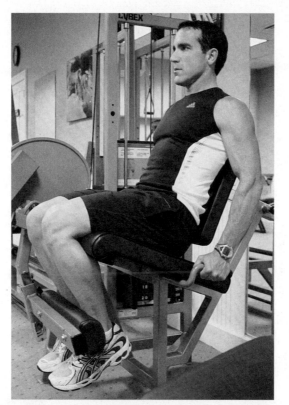

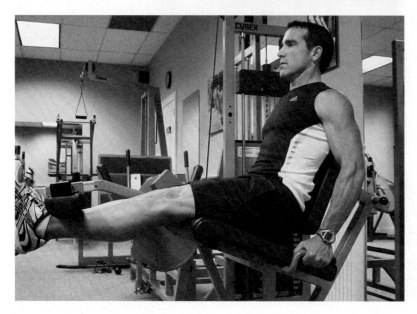

With the pad resting just above your ankles, extend both legs until your legs are straight. Hold for one count, then slowly lower.

Single-Leg Machine Leg Extension

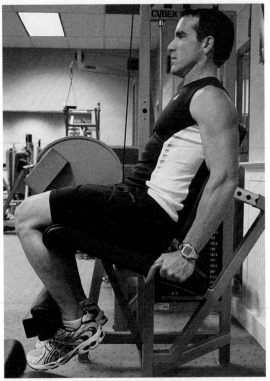

The same exercise, one leg at a time.

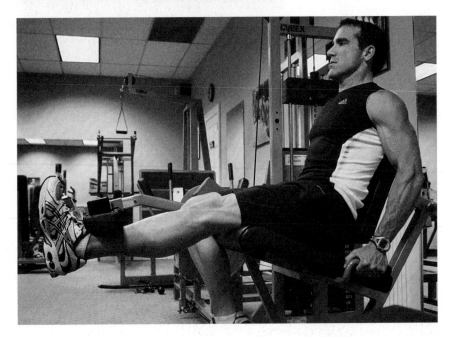

Machine Leg Abduction

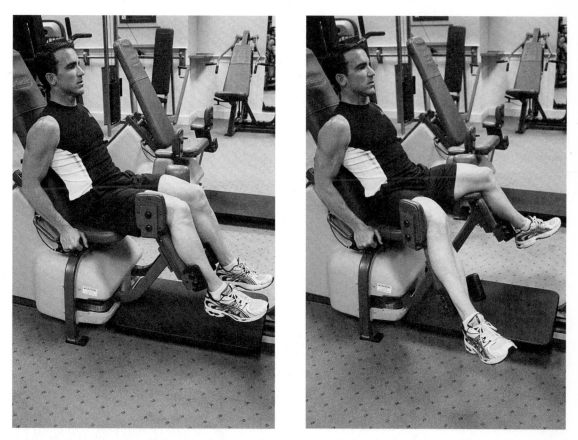

Open your legs and press the pads away from your body, hold for 1 second, then slowly return to the starting position.

Machine Leg Adduction

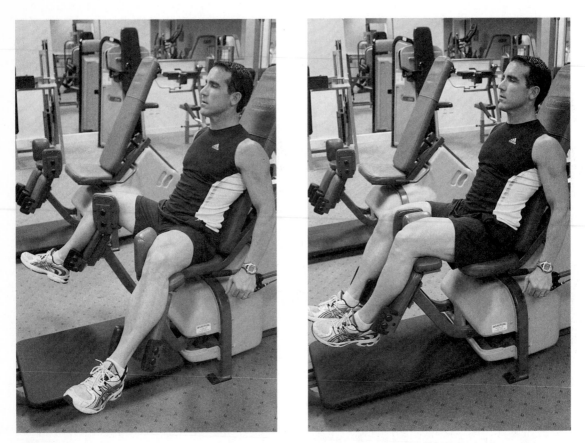

Close your legs and press the pads together, hold for 1 second, then slowly return to the starting position.

Machine Chest Press

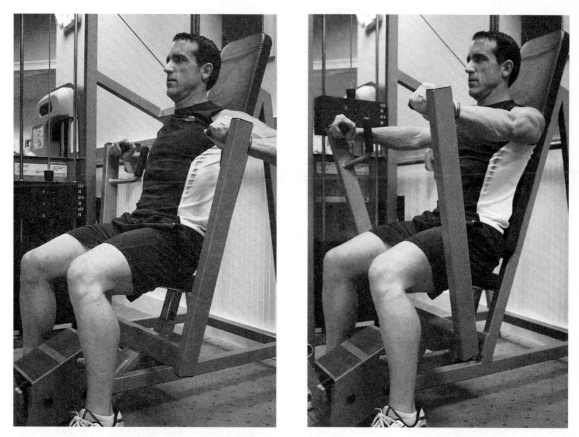

Keeping your shoulders down and neck relaxed, push the handles away from your body until your arms are extended, hold for 1 second, then slowly return to the starting position.

Machine Leg Press

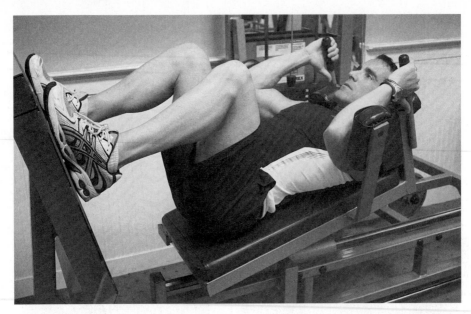

Your feet should be a little wider than shoulder-width apart. Keeping your knees behind your toes, lower your body down to just above 90 degrees of knee bend. Hold for 1 second, then extend your legs and return to the starting position.

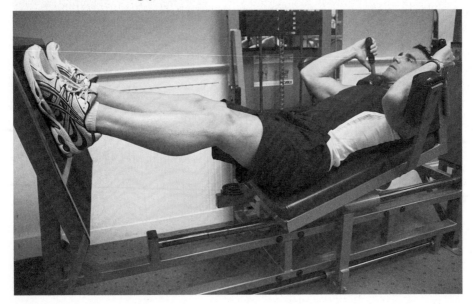

Single-Leg Machine Leg Press

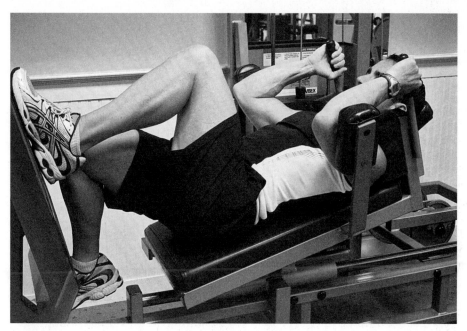

The same exercise, one leg at a time.

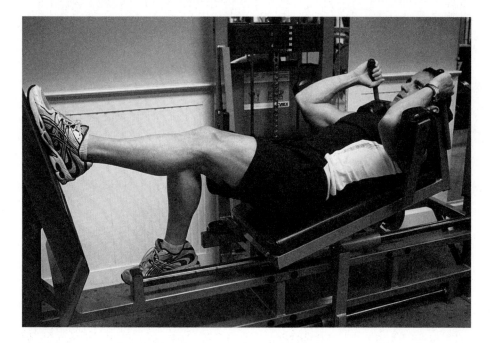

Calf Raise in Leg Press Machine

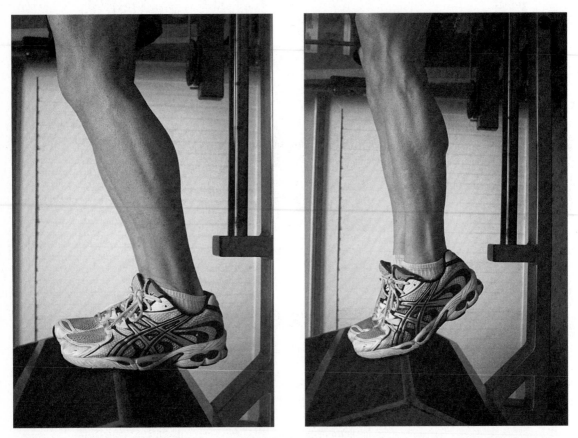

While in the leg press machine, position your feet so that your toes are on the bottom of the footrest. With your legs extended, drop your heels a few inches, then press on your toes and raise your body as high as you can.

Single-Leg Calf Raise in Leg Press Machine

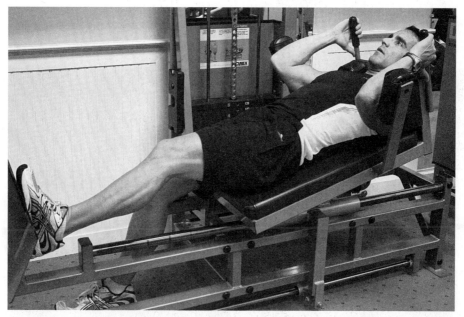

The same exercise, but with less weight and doing one calf at a time.

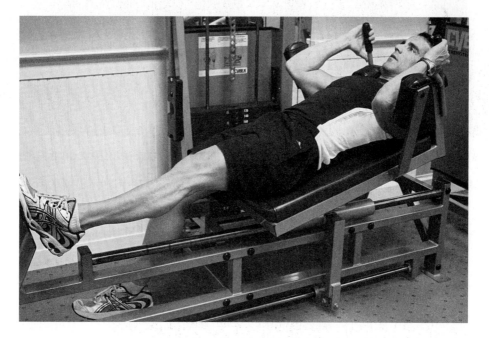

Machine Chest Fly

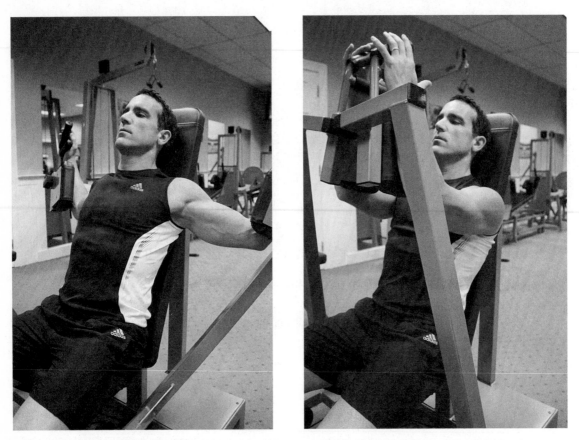

Press the pads together until they touch lightly, hold for 1 second, then slowly return to the starting position.

Machine Incline Chest Press

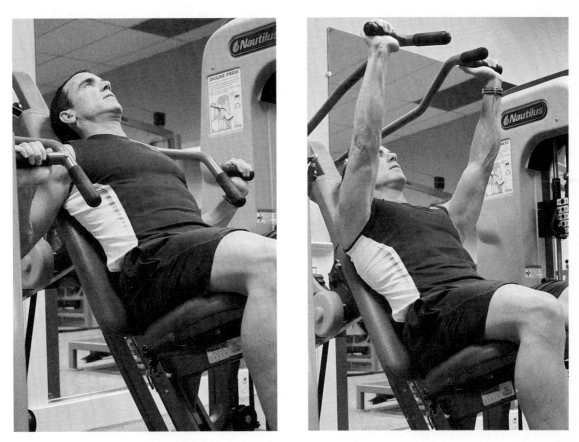

Push the handles away from your body until your arm are extended, hold for 1 second, then slowly return to the starting position.

Machine Seated Leg Curl

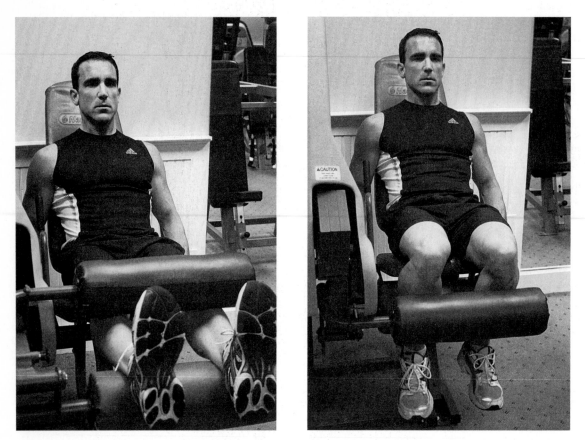

Slowly pull the pad under you toward your butt, hold for 1 second, then slowly return to the starting position.

Machine Triceps Extension

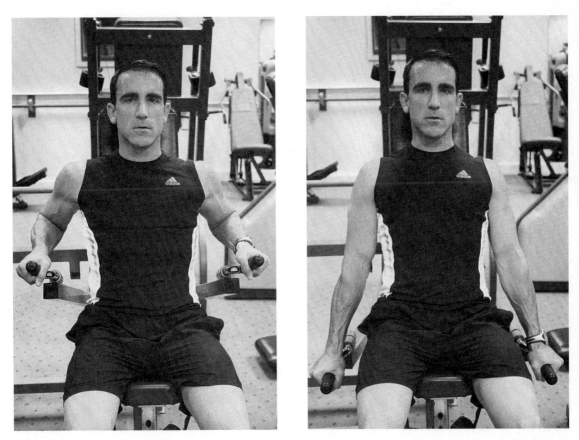

Press the handles until your arms are fully extended, hold for 1 second, then slowly return to the starting position.

Machine-Assisted Triceps Dip

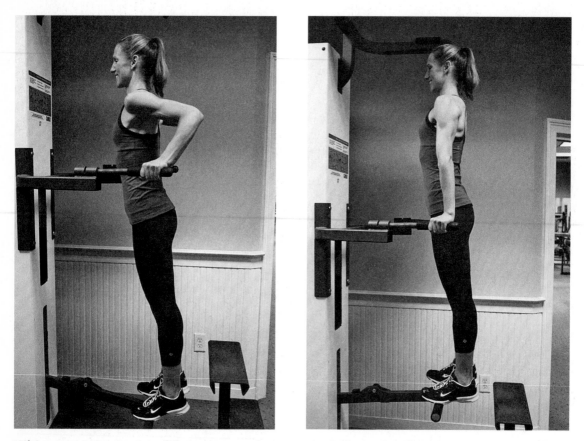

With your arms bent to 90 degrees, raise your body by extending your arms until they are straight. Hold for 1 second, then slowly lower to the starting position.

Machine-Assisted Pull-up

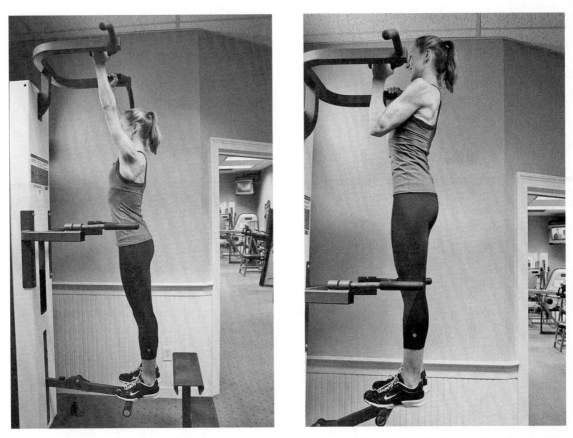

Holding firmly on to the handles, pull your body up until your head clears the bar, hold for 1 second, then slowly lower.

Machine Biceps Curl

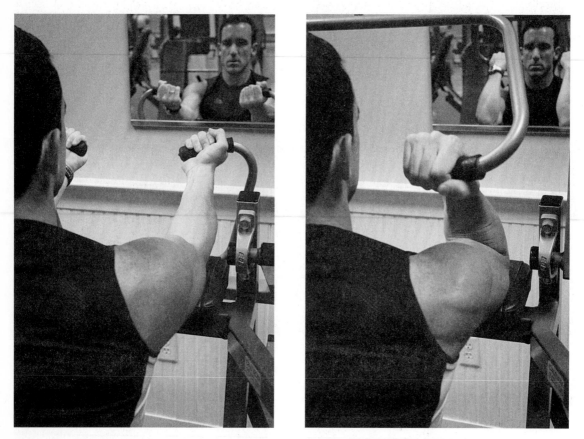

Bring the handles toward your shoulders, hold for 1 second, then slowly lower them until your arms are almost fully extended. Repeat.

Single-Arm Machine Biceps Curl

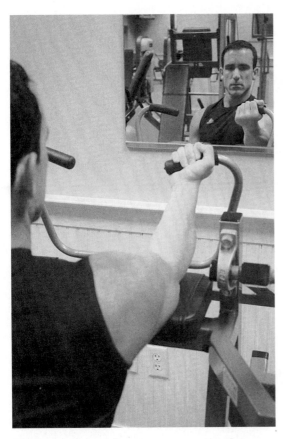 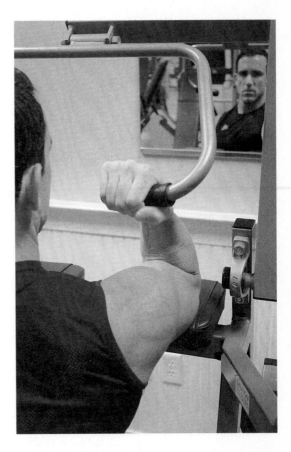

The same exercise, one arm at a time.

Machine Lat Pull-down, Wide Bar, Prone Grip

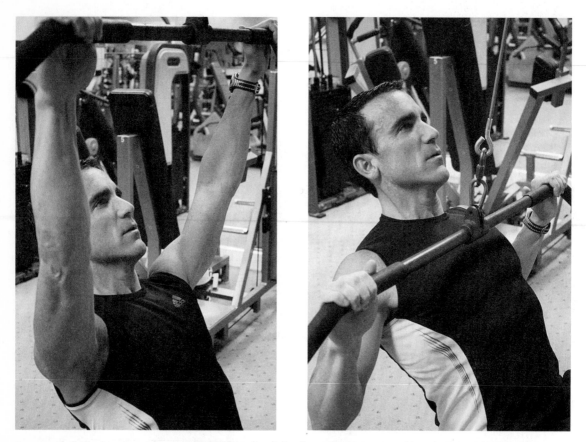

Lean slightly back while holding the straight bar above you with your hands facing away from you and slightly more than shoulder-width apart. Initiating the movement from your back, keep your chest out and pull the bar to the middle of your chest, pressing your shoulder blades together. Hold for 1 second, then slowly raise the bar.

Machine Lat Pull-down, Close Grip

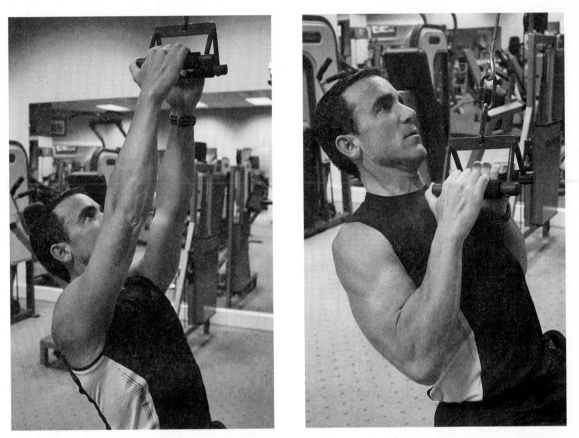

Lean slightly back while holding the close-grip attachment above you. Initiating the movement from your back, keep your chest out while pulling the handles to the middle of your chest, pressing your shoulder blades together. Hold for 1 second, then slowly raise the handles.

Machine Lat Pull-down, Wide Bar, Supine Grip

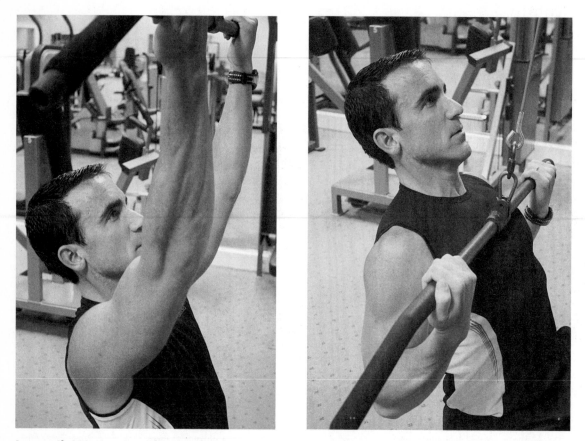

Lean slightly back while holding the straight bar above you with your hands shoulder-width apart and your palms facing you. Initiating the movement from your back, keep your chest out and pull the bar to the middle of your chest, pressing your shoulder blades together. Hold for 1 second, then slowly raise the bar.

Machine Lat Pull-down, Rope

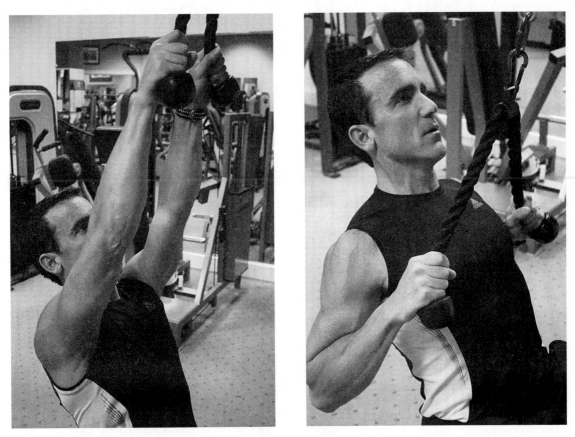

Lean slightly back while holding the rope attachment above you. Initiating the movement from your back, keep your chest out while pulling the rope down to either side of your chest, pressing your shoulder blades together. Hold for 1 second, then slowly raise the rope.

Smith Machine Squat

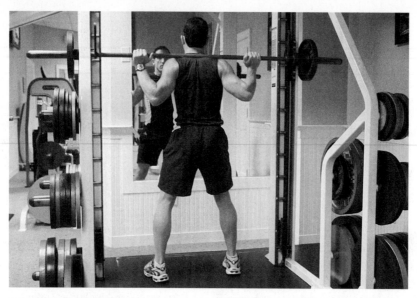

Stand in the Smith machine with your feet a little more than shoulder-width apart and your toes pointing forward, resting the bar on your shoulders behind your head. Keeping your chest up and your knees behind your toes, lower your body to just above 90 degrees of knee bend. Hold for 1 second, then return to the starting position.

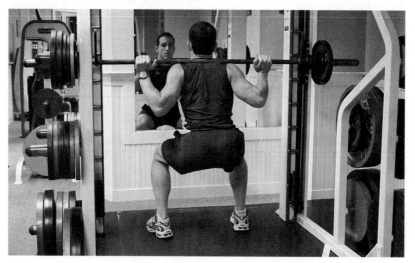

Smith Machine Lunge

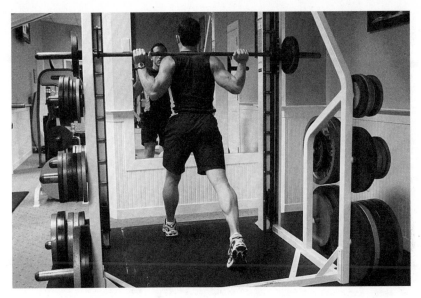

Stand in the Smith machine with one foot forward and one back, resting the bar on your shoulders behind your head. Keeping your chest up and your knees behind your toes, lower your body straight to the floor until your back knee is almost touching the floor, hold for 1 second, then rise to the starting position.

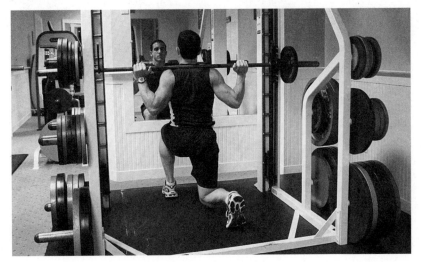

Smith Machine Calf Raise

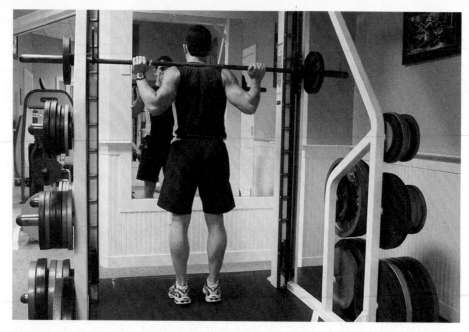

Stand in the Smith machine with your feet an inch or two apart, resting the bar on your shoulders behind your head. Pressing down on

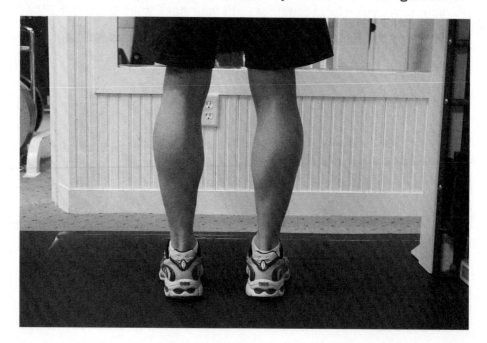

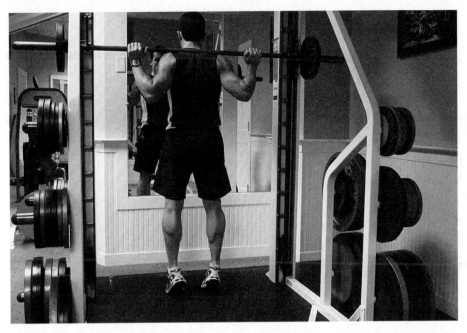

your toes, lift your heels off the ground and raise your body, hold for 1 second, then lower to the starting position.

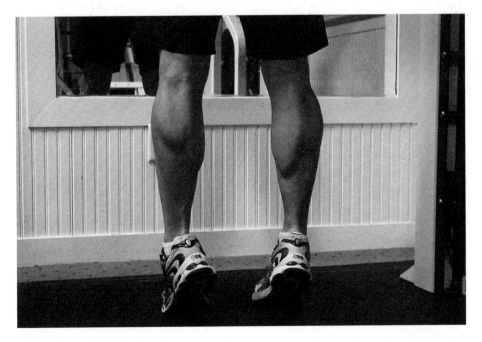

Plate-Loaded Machines

There are no weight stacks built into these machines; you have to physically load plates on them. Because they require changing heavy plates, these machines are better suited to stronger people.

Though the way you load the weight may be different between selectorized and plate-loaded machines, the basic movements and muscles targeted remain the same. So a chest press in a selectorized machine would be the same basic exercise as a chest press in a plate-loaded machine. For the purposes of this book, when a workout calls for a machine exercise such as a biceps curl, you have the option of using either type. As it would be redundant to illustrate all of the same variations of both types of machines, refer to the selectorized machine photos when choosing a plate-loaded machine. Just remember to mix up the exercises!

Lifting Lingo: Circuit training

Circuit training involves performing a series of exercises in a certain order with little rest in between. The constant movement keeps the heart rate elevated, adding a cardiovascular component to the strength program. It is an extremely efficient way for many people to work out, especially those who have limited time in the gym.

Sample Strength Circuit

You can perform circuits with any type of equipment. Machines, free weights, body weight, cables, or a mixture of all of these. The thing to remember is to keep moving quickly and to target the entire body whenever possible. Work your body from head to toe. You will be shocked at how fast you can get your workout in when you do circuit training. Make no mistake about it: there is nothing magical about sixty-minute workouts. Remember to focus on quality, not quantity. By doing circuit training you can work your entire body and be in and out of the gym in thirty minutes or less. Check out two great circuits on pages 269 and 275.

The following exercises should be done using any mix of the machines:

- Chest press
- Back row

- Shoulder press
- Triceps press
- Biceps curl
- Leg extension
- Leg curl
- Leg press
- Abdominal curl
- Back extension

This group of exercises, when performed one after the other, is extremely simple yet extremely effective. It hits all the major muscle groups. You should do twelve repetitions of each with no rest in between, making sure the weights are challenging on the last few repetitions. You can do one to three full circuits, depending on the time you have available.

Free Weights

These include dumbbells, barbells, kettlebells, and so on. It's the "freedom" of free weights that defines what they are: you have complete freedom of movement and the freedom to do an infinite number of exercises with them. Freedom is both good and bad.

GOOD: They force you to use more muscles. They help develop your balance and coordination. They are more "functional" than machines, strengthening us for both daily life and sports.

BAD: You need to know what exercises to do and how to do them. There is much more freedom to do exercises incorrectly. There is also a much greater chance of injury when using free weights.

The freedom of movement challenges more muscles of your body, as you are forced to balance and control the weights in space.

Dumbbell Deadlift

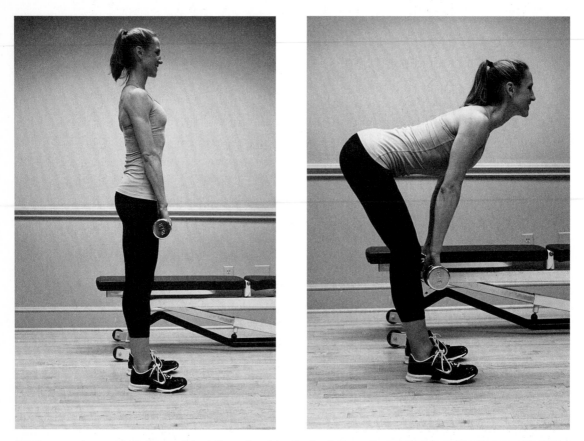

With your legs straight and holding dumbbells in front of your thighs, slowly bend at the waist and lower the weights toward the floor, keeping your shoulders back and your back flat. When you can go no farther without rounding your back, hold for 1 second, then slowly rise.

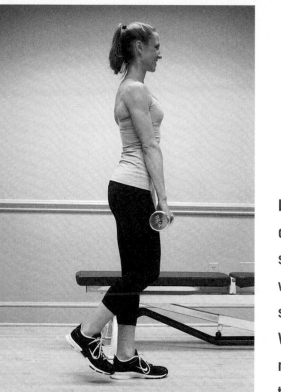

Single-Leg Dumbbell Deadlift

Balancing on one leg and holding dumbbells in front of your thighs, slowly bend at the waist and lower the weights toward the floor, keeping your shoulders back and your back flat. When you can go no farther without rounding your back, hold for 1 second, then slowly rise.

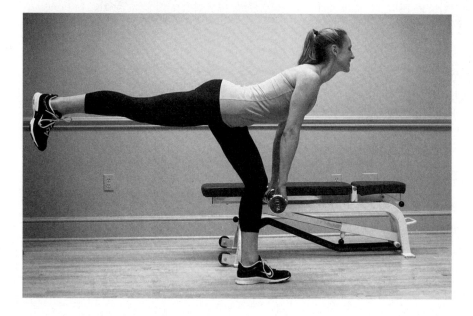

Dumbbell Row

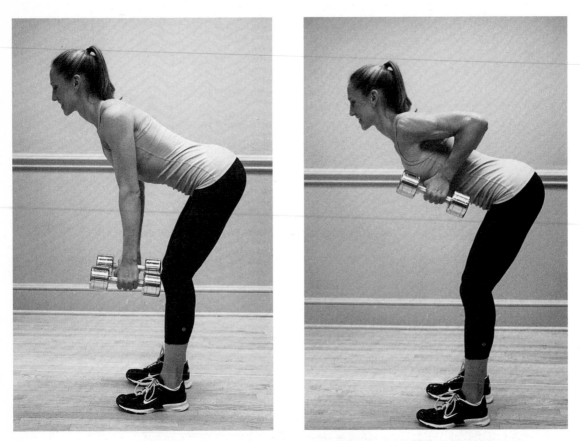

Bend at the waist with your upper body as parallel as possible to the floor and your back flat, not rounded. With your arms straight down and holding dumbbells, pull them up toward your body, hold for 1 second, then lower them.

Single-Arm Dumbbell Row

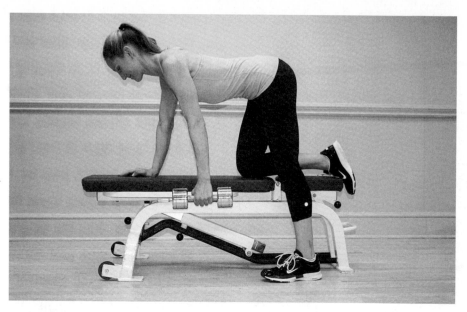

Rest with one knee and one arm on a bench, holding a dumbbell, with the other arm extended down toward the floor. Keeping your upper body as parallel as possible to the floor and your back flat, not rounded, pull the weight up toward your body, hold for 1 second, then lower it.

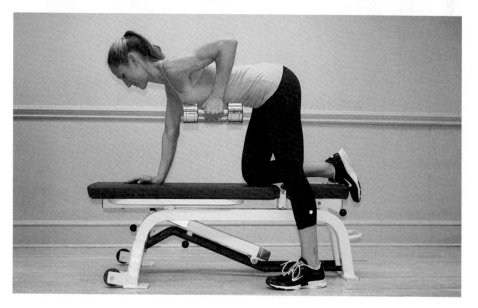

Dumbbell Front and Side Raise

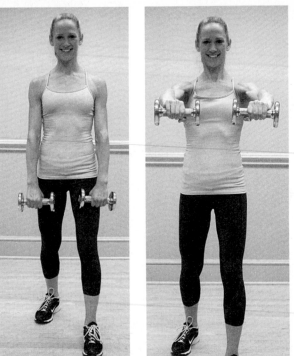

Stand in a split stance with one foot in front of the other and your knees slightly bent. Holding the dumbbells against your waist with your elbows slightly bent, slowly raise them in front of you to shoulder height, hold for 1 second, then slowly lower them. Next, slowly raise the weights out to your sides with your elbows slightly bent, up to shoulder height, hold for 1 second, then lower them to the starting position.

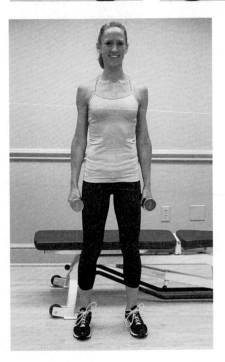

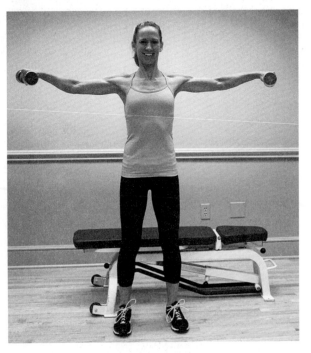

Dumbbell Side Raise

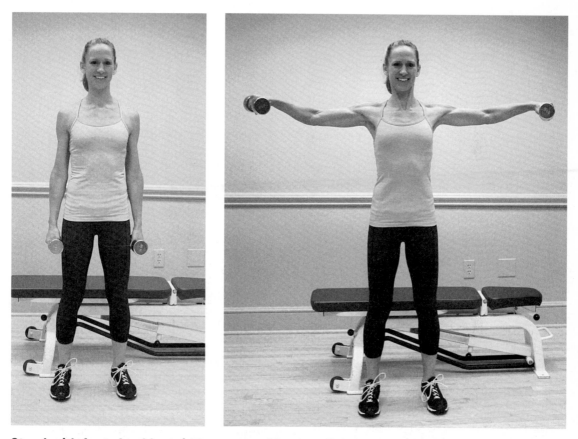

Stand with feet shoulder-width apart and knees slightly bent. Holding the dumbbells at your sides with your elbows slightly bent, slowly raise them out to your sides, keeping your elbows slightly bent, up to shoulder height, hold for 1 second, then lower back to starting position.

Dumbbell Shoulder Press

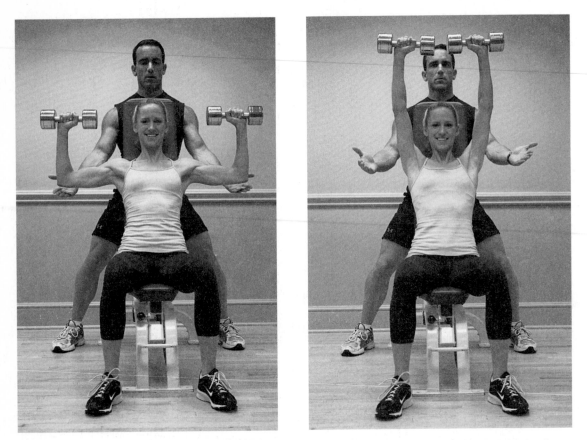

Hold dumbbells up with your elbows in line with your shoulders and your palms facing forward. Press them over your head until the ends are almost touching, then slowly lower them to the starting position.

Dumbbell Rear Delt Fly

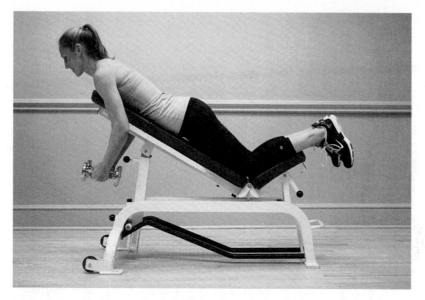

Lie facedown on an incline, holding dumbbells underneath you with your palms facing. Keeping your back flat, raise the weights out to the side with a slight bend in your elbows until they are in line with your shoulders, hold for 1 second, then lower back down.

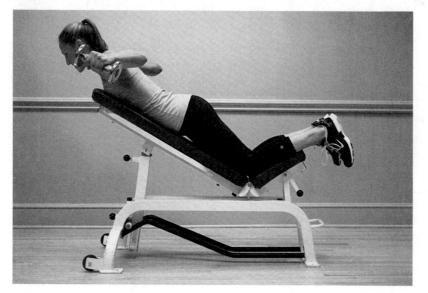

Flat-Bench Barbell Chest Press

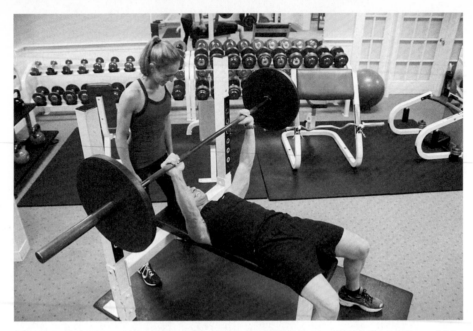

Lie on a flat bench holding a barbell slightly more than shoulder-width apart. Slowly lower the bar until it is a few inches from your chest, then press it back up until your arms are fully extended.

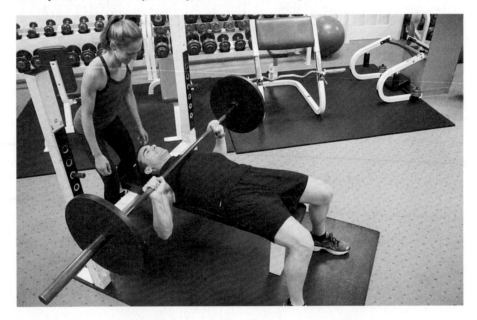

Incline Dumbbell Chest Press

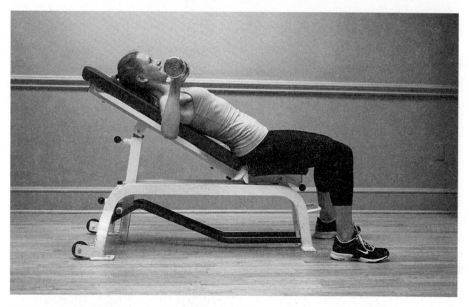

Lie on an incline bench holding dumbbells slightly wider than shoulder-width apart. Press them up until your arms are fully extended, then lower them back to the starting position.

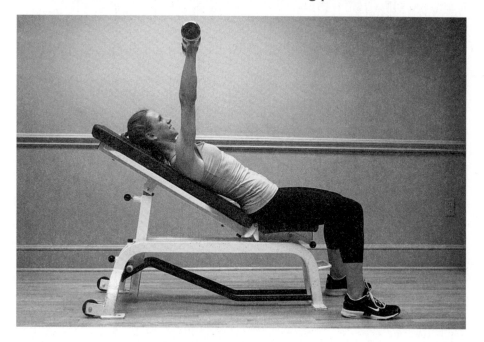

Incline Barbell Bench Press

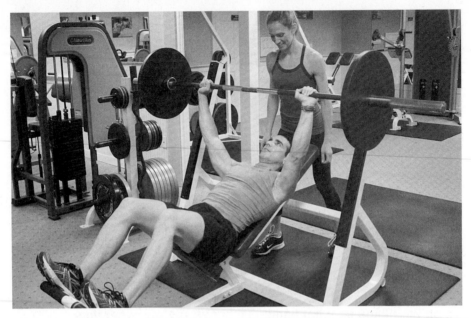

Lie on an incline bench holding a barbell slightly more than shoulder-width apart. Slowly lower the bar until it is a few inches from your chest, then press it back up until your arms are fully extended.

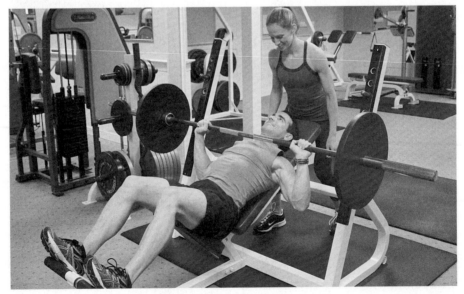

Dumbbell Chest Fly

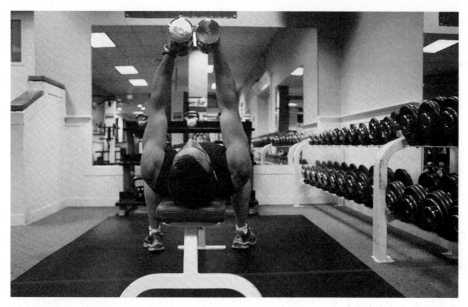

Lie on your back on a flat bench, holding dumbbells over your chest with your palms facing. With your elbows slightly bent, slowly lower the weights out to the sides until they are just above your body. Hold for 1 second, then raise them back to the starting position.

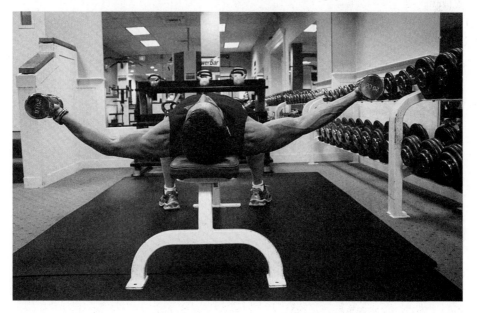

Flat-Bench Dumbbell Chest Press

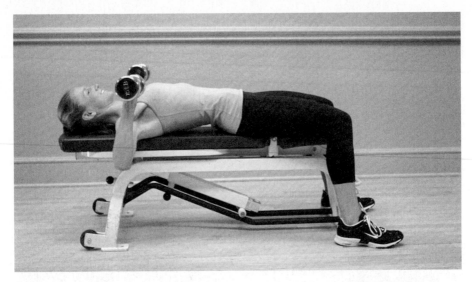

Lie on a flat bench holding dumbbells with your arms bent to 90 degrees and your palms facing away from you. Press the weights up and over your chest until the ends are almost touching, then slowly lower them.

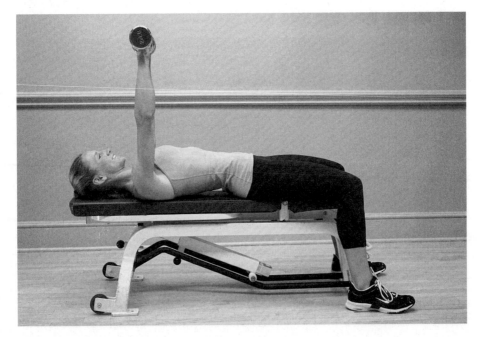

Barbell Row

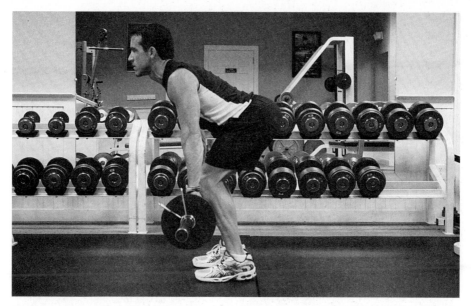

Bend at the waist with your upper body as parallel as possible to the floor and your back flat, not rounded. Holding a barbell under your chest with your arms straight down, pull it up toward your body, hold for 1 second, then lower it.

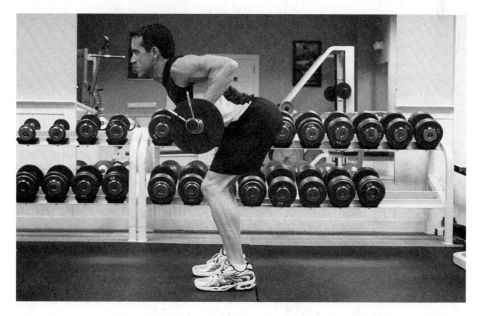

Barbell Biceps Curl

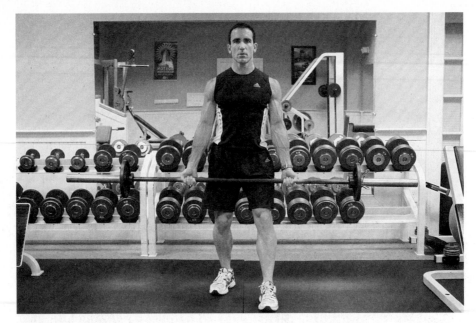

Hold a barbell in front of your thighs with your palms facing up. Slowly raise the barbell toward your shoulders, hold for 1 second, then slowly lower it.

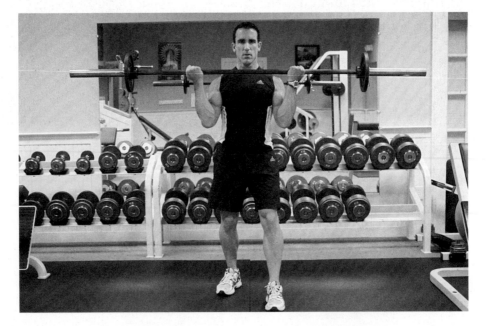

Preacher Bench Bar: Biceps Curl

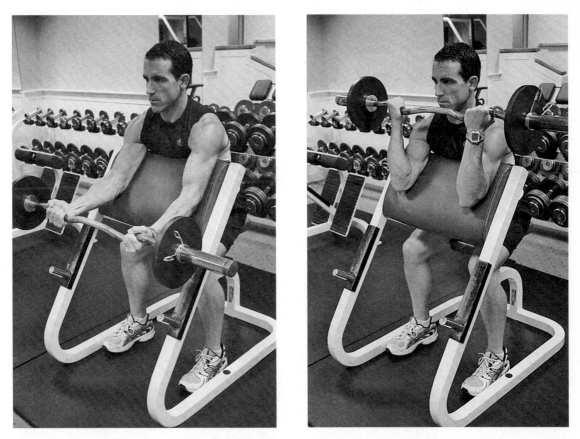

Sit on the preacher bench holding the curl bar with your hands roughly shoulder-width apart. Slowly raise the bar toward your shoulders, hold for 1 second, then slowly lower it.

Preacher Bench Dumbbell Biceps Curl

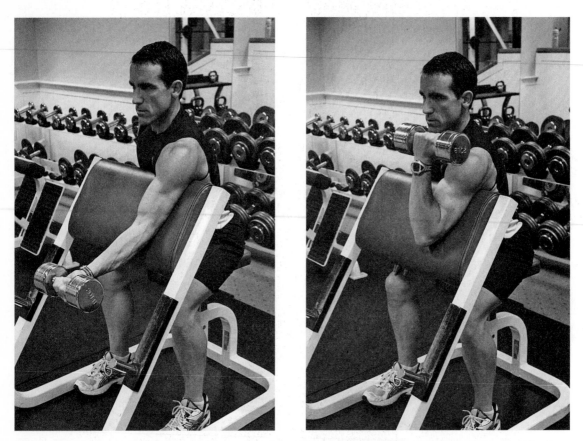

Sit on the preacher bench holding a dumbbell in one hand. Slowly raise the dumbbell toward your shoulder, hold for 1 second, then slowly lower it back down.

Barbell Reverse Curl

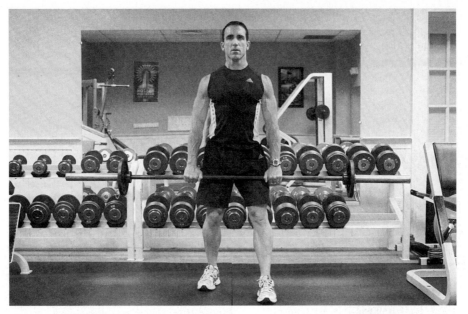

Hold a barbell in front of your thighs with your palms facing down. Slowly raise the barbell up toward your shoulders, hold for 1 second, then slowly lower it.

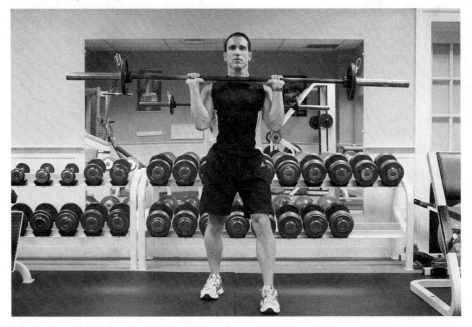

Dumbbell Biceps Curl

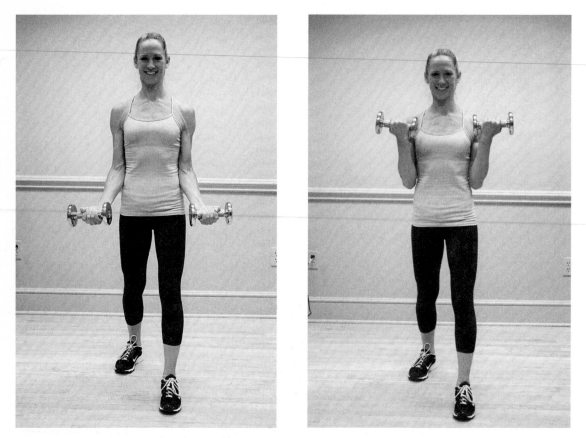

Hold dumbbells with your elbows tucked in to your sides and your palms facing forward. Slowly raise the weights toward your shoulders, hold for 1 second, then slowly lower them.

Dumbbell Triceps Kickback

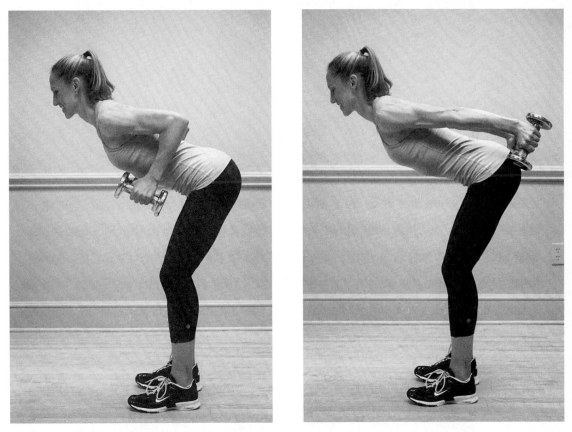

Holding dumbbells, bend over until your upper body is as parallel to the floor as possible. Bring your elbows up so that your upper arms are parallel to the floor. With your palms facing toward you, extend the weights back and up until your arms are fully extended, hold for 1 second, then slowly lower them. Do not move your upper arms throughout the exercise.

Single-Arm Dumbbell Triceps Kickback

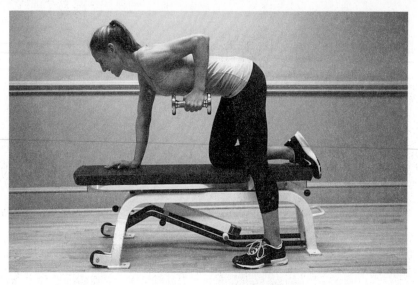

Place one arm and one knee on a bench for balance while holding a dumbbell in the other hand. Position your upper body so that it is parallel to the floor and bring your elbow up so that your upper arm is parallel to the floor. With your palm facing toward you, extend the weight back and up until your arm is fully extended, hold for 1 second, then slowly lower it. Do not move your upper arm throughout the exercise.

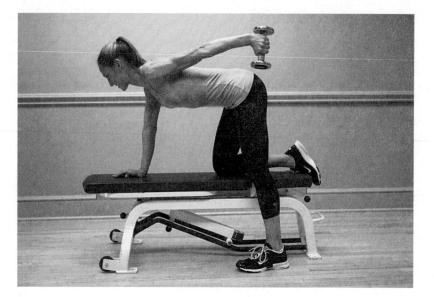

Flat-Bench Close-Grip Triceps Bench Press

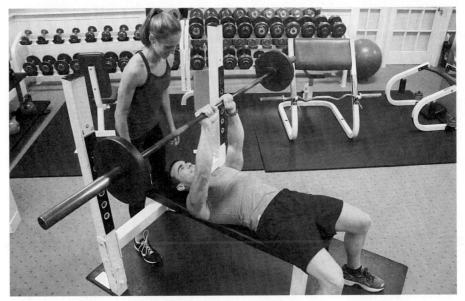

Lie on a flat bench holding a barbell above you with your hands a few inches apart. Slowly lower the barbell until it is a few inches from your chest, then press it up until your arms are fully extended.

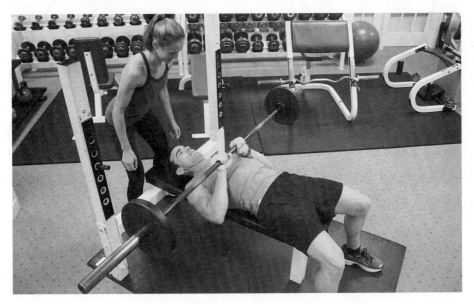

Dumbbell Squat

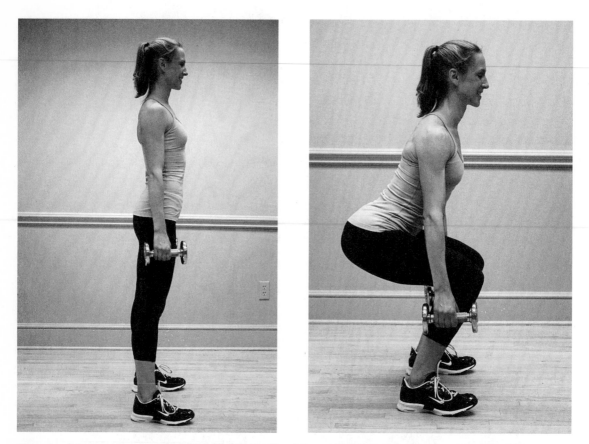

Stand with your feet a little wider than shoulder-width apart and your toes pointing forward, holding a pair of dumbbells at your sides. Keeping your chest up and your knees behind your toes, lower your body to just above 90 degrees of knee bend. Hold for 1 second, then return to the starting position.

Single-Leg Ball Squat

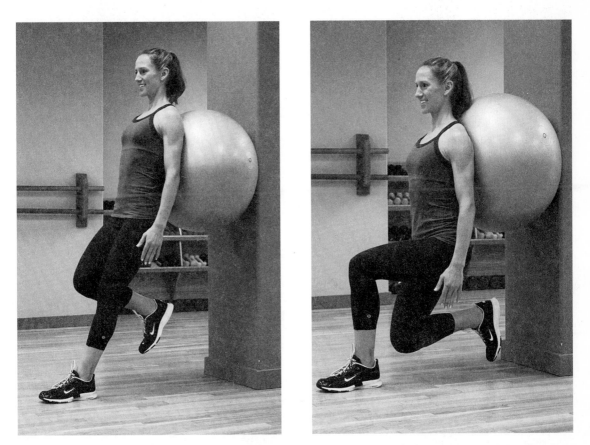

Stand on one leg while pressing a stability ball into a wall with your back. Keeping your chest up and your knees behind your toes, lower your body to just above 90 degrees of knee bend, hold for 1 second, then return to the starting position.

Dumbbell Ball Squat

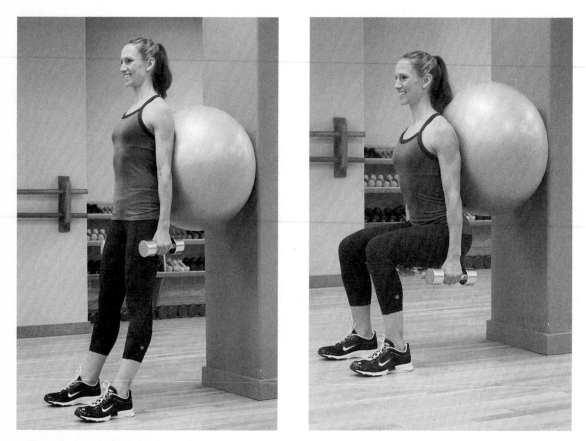

Stand holding dumbbells at your sides while pressing a stability ball into a wall with your back. Your feet should be a little wider than shoulder-width apart with your toes pointing forward. Keeping your chest up and your knees behind your toes, lower your body to just above 90 degrees of knee bend and hold for 1 second, then return to the starting position.

Dumbbell Forward Lunge

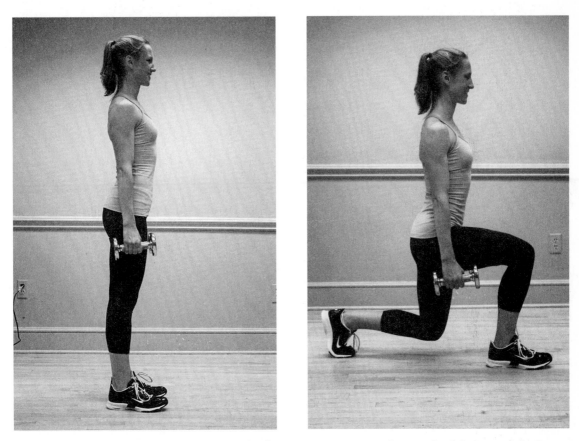

Keep your chest up and your knees behind your toes, step forward with your right leg until your left knee is a few inches off the floor. Hold for 1 second, step back, then repeat with your left leg.

Dumbbell Walking Lunge

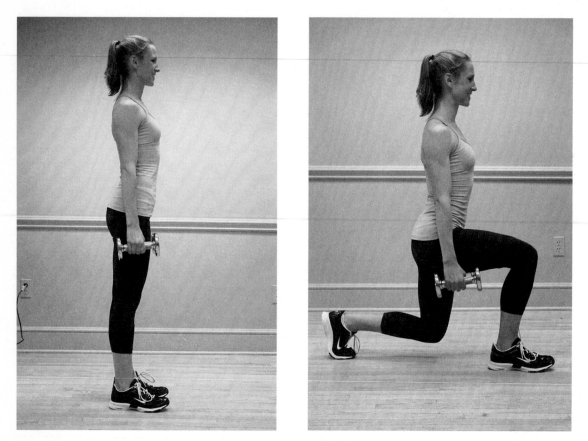

Keeping your chest up and your knees behind your toes, walk across the gym while holding a set of dumbbells, slowly lowering your body straight to the floor until your back knee is almost touching the floor, holding for 1 second, then repeating with the other leg.

Dumbbell Stationary Lunge

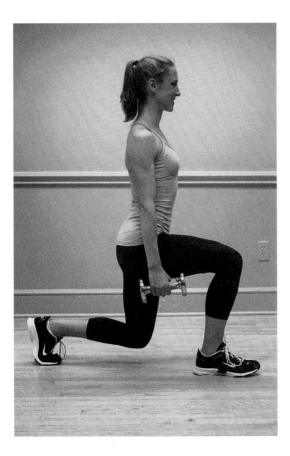

Stand in a split stance with one leg forward and one back, holding a pair of dumbbells at your sides. Keep your chest up and your knees behind your toes, lower your body straight to the floor until your back knee is almost touching the floor. Hold for 1 second, then return to the starting position.

Dumbbell Bench Step-up

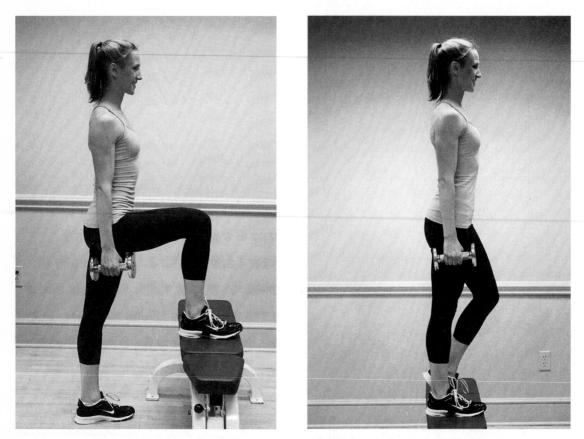

Place your right foot on a bench about knee height while holding dumbbells at your sides. Step up and tap your left foot on the bench while fully extending your right leg, slowly step back down with the left leg, then immediately repeat.

Barbell Deadlift

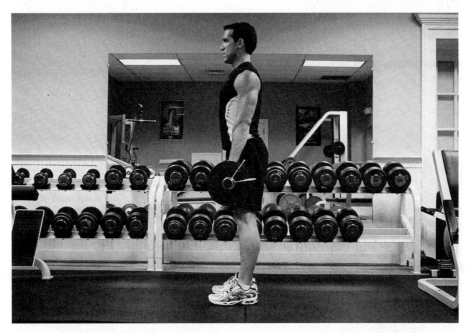

With your legs straight and holding a barbell in front of your thighs, slowly bend at the waist and lower the weights toward the floor, keeping your shoulders back and your back flat. When you can go no farther without rounding your back, hold for 1 second, then slowly rise.

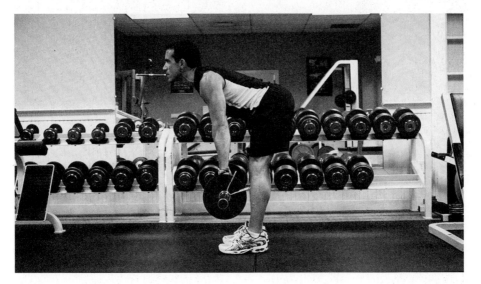

Barbell Lunge

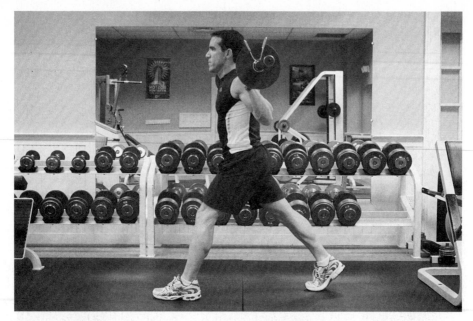

With a barbell resting on your shoulders behind your head, step forward with your left leg until your right knee is a few inches off the floor, making sure to keep your chest up and your knee behind your toes. Hold for 1 second, step back, then repeat with your right leg.

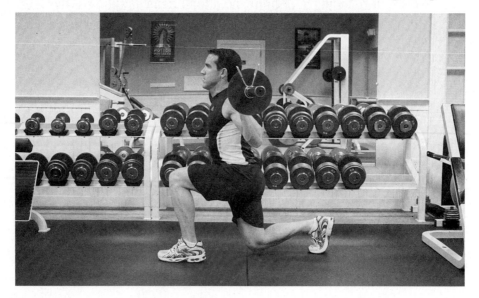

Ball Squat with Dumbbell Biceps Curl

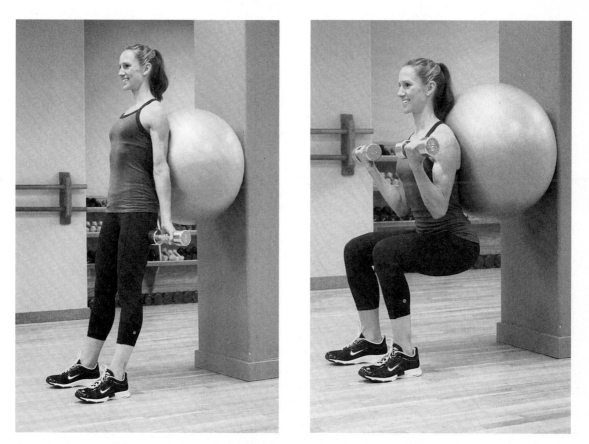

Stand with your feet a little more than shoulder-width apart and your toes pointing forward, holding a pair of dumbbells at your sides. Keeping your chest up and your knees behind your toes, lower your body to just above 90 degrees of knee bend while bringing the weights up toward your shoulders. Hold for 1 second, then return to the starting position.

Ball Squat with Dumbbell Shoulder Press

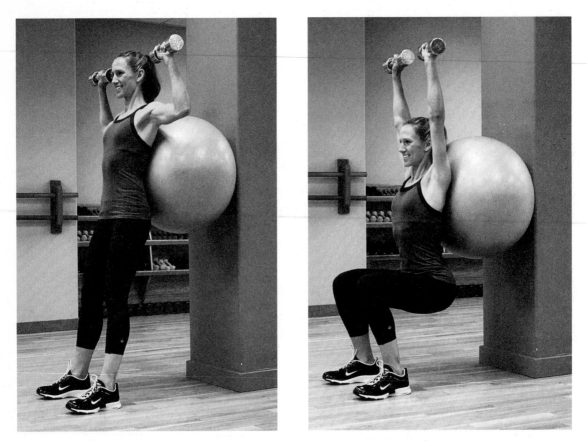

Stand with your feet a little more than shoulder-width apart and your toes pointing forward, holding a pair of dumbbells at above your shoulders with your palms facing forward. Keeping your chest up and your knees behind your toes, lower your body to just above 90 degrees of knee bend while pressing the weights up over your head until they are almost touching. Hold for 1 second, then return to the starting position.

Body-Weight Exercises

A subcategory of free-weight exercises is body-weight exercises. Many of the exercises that can be done with free weights can also be performed using just your own body weight. In fact, one of the ways I progress my clients is to begin with basic body-weight exercises and then add additional resistance when appropriate. Remember that body-weight exercises are some of the most effective for transforming your body. They can be performed anywhere: at home, while on vacation, outside, and so on.

Body-weight exercises are extremely functional. They help strengthen your body for the activities of daily living, as well as any sports you might play. We squat, lunge, and push-up every day. The stronger and better we are at performing these basic movements, the better our quality of life will be. It will be more enjoyable, and we will be injured less often.

A natural progression from doing body-weight exercises is to use free weights. Like body-weight exercises, free weights also challenge our muscles in a functional manner. By training with them we will strengthen our bodies even further, increase our lean muscle mass, and boost our metabolism.

Here are a few of the best body-weight moves:

Push-up

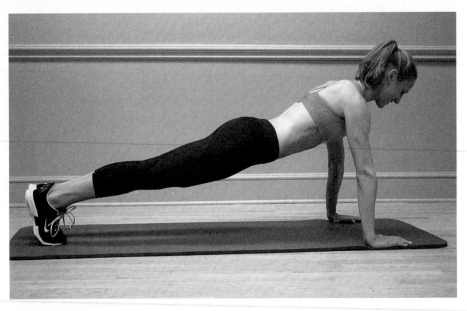

Holding your body up in a straight line on your hands (just slightly more than shoulder-width apart) and your toes, lower slowly until your chest is a few inches off the floor, then return to the starting position. Beginners may start on their knees.

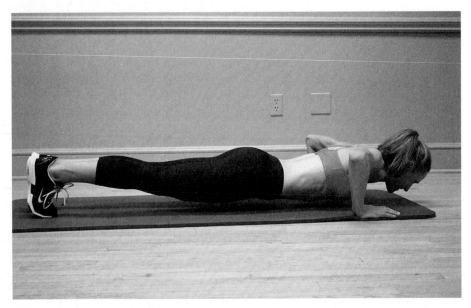

Ball Push-up

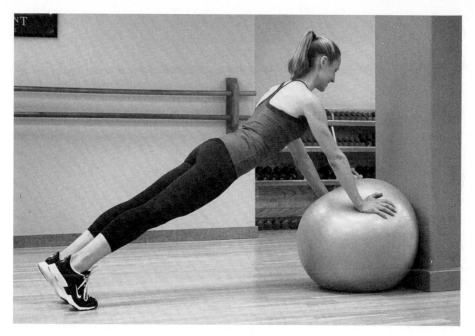

Holding your body in a straight line with your hands on a stability ball pressed against a wall, lower slowly until your chest is a few inches off the ball, then return to the starting position.

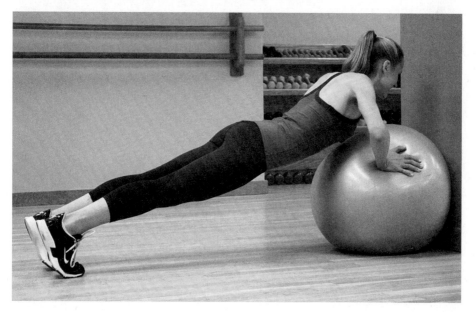

Decline Push-up

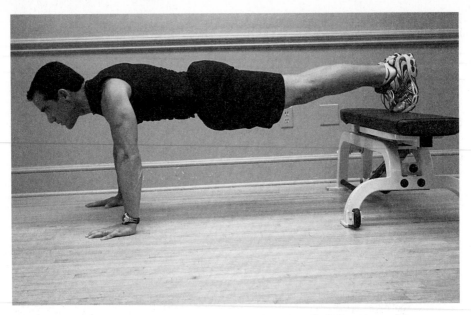

With your toes up on a bench and your hands slightly more than shoulder-width apart on the floor, lower slowly until your chest is a few inches off of the floor, then return to the starting position.

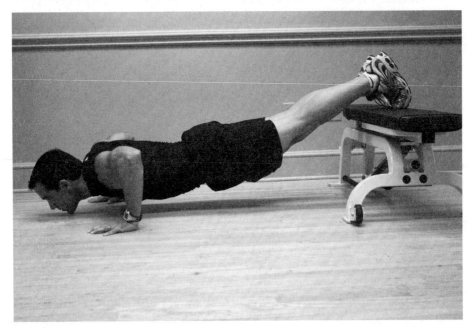

Incline Push-up

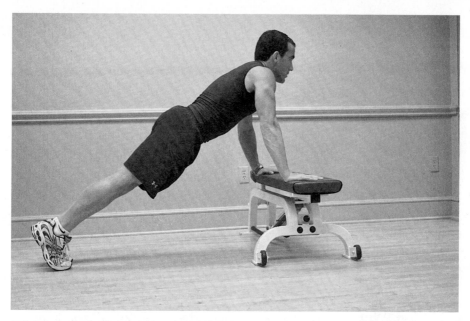

With your toes on the floor and your hands slightly more than shoulder-width apart on a bench, lower slowly until your chest is a few inches off the bench, then return to the starting position.

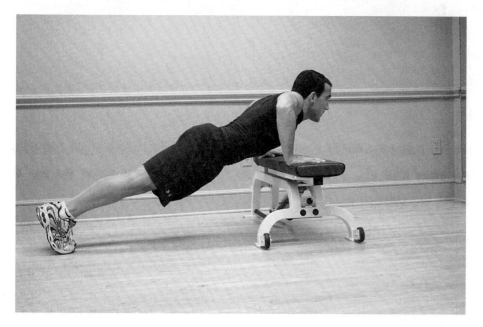

Pull-up

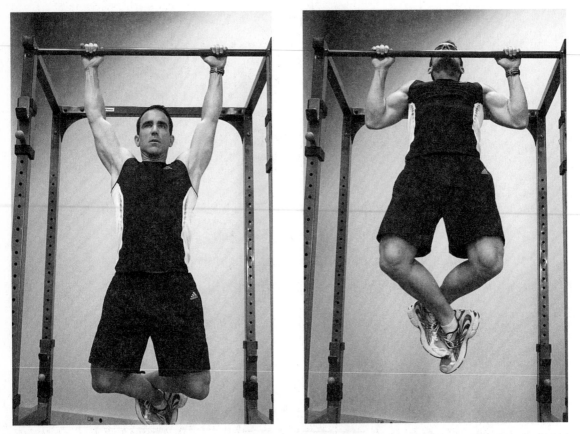

Hang from a bar with your hands slightly more than shoulder-width apart and your palms facing away from you. Pull your body up until your head is above the bar, then slowly lower to the starting position.

Chin-up

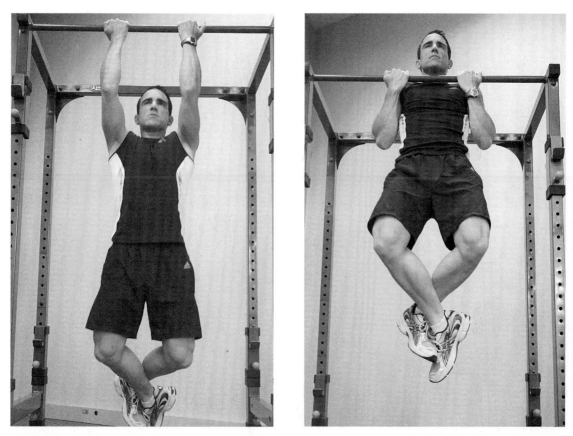

Hang from a bar with your hands shoulder-width apart and your palms facing you. Pull your body up until your head is above the bar, then slowly lower to the starting position.

Dip

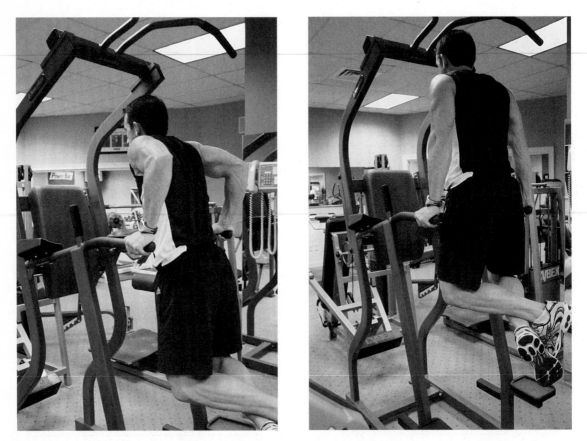

In a dip station, hold your body up with your arms bent to 90 degrees. Raise your body until your arms are fully extended, then slowly lower to the starting position.

Bench Dip

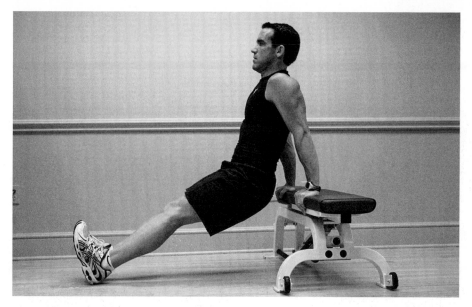

Position yourself on the side of a bench with your back to it, holding yourself up with your hands on the edge. Slowly bend your elbows and lower your body to several inches from the floor, hold for 1 second, then raise your body until your arms are fully extended.

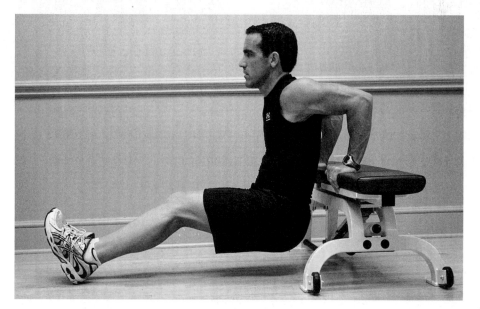

Walking Lunge

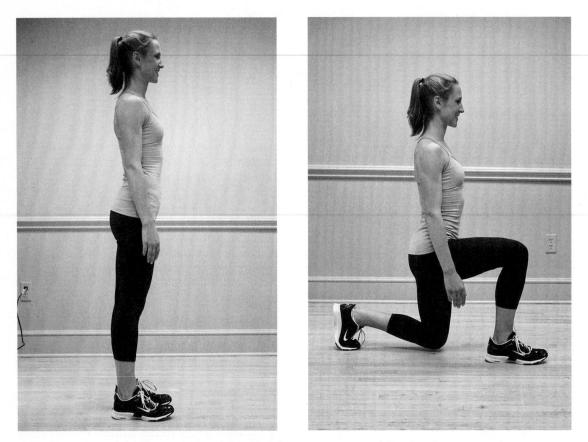

Keeping your chest up and your knee behind your toes, walk slowly across the gym. With each stride, lower your body straight to the floor until your back knee is almost touching the floor, pause, and repeat with the other leg.

Stationary Lunge

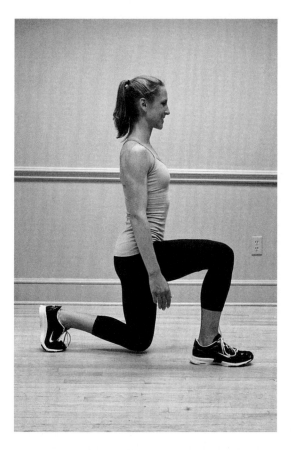

Stand in a split stance with one foot forward and one back. Keeping your chest up and your knee behind your toes, lower your body straight to the floor until your back knee is almost touching the floor. Hold for 1 second, then return to the starting position.

Bench Step-up

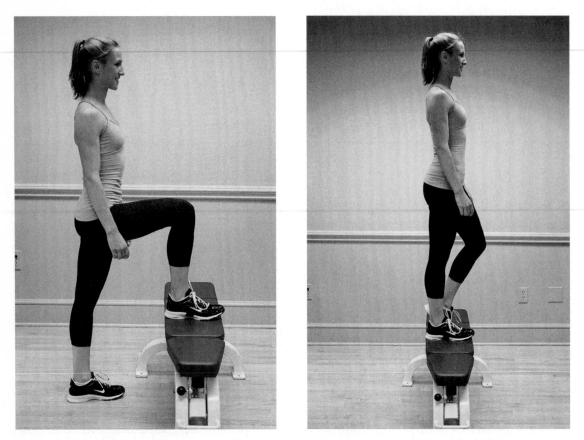

Place your right foot on a bench about knee height. Step up and tap your left foot on the bench while fully extending your right leg, slowly step back down with the left leg, then immediately repeat.

Ball Hamstring Curl

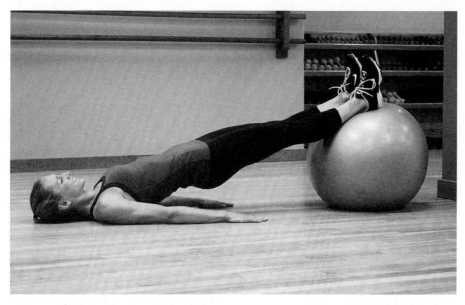

With your heels up on a stability ball, your shoulders on the floor, and your body held up off the floor in a straight line, pull the ball to your butt, then return to the starting position. Do not allow your hips to touch the floor throughout the exercise.

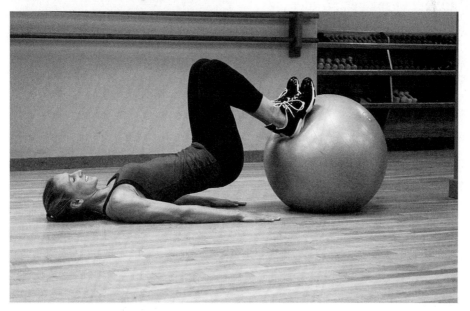

Stability Ball Wall Sit

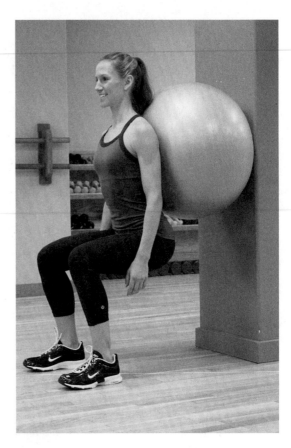

Stand, pressing a stability ball into a wall with your back. Your feet should be a little more than shoulder-width apart with your toes pointing forward. Keeping your chest up and your knees behind your toes, lower your body to just above 90 degrees of knee bend and hold for the prescribed amount of time, then return to the starting position.

Ball Squat

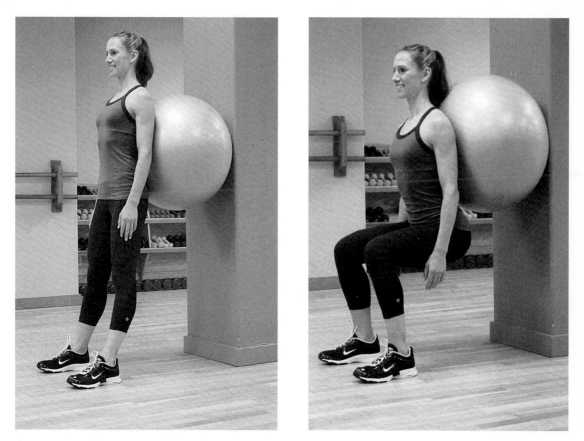

Stand, pressing a stability ball into a wall with your back. Your feet should be a little more than shoulder-width apart with your toes pointing forward. Keeping your chest up and your knees behind your toes, lower your body to just above 90 degrees of knee bend, hold for 1 second, then return to the starting position.

BOSU Squat

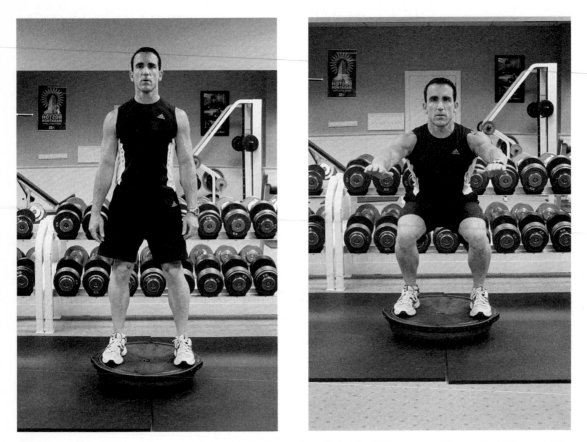

Stand on a **BOSU** balance trainer. Your feet should be a little more than shoulder-width apart with your toes pointing forward. Keeping your chest up and your knees behind your toes, lower your body to just above 90 degrees of knee bend, hold for 1 second, then return to the starting position.

Balance Board Squat

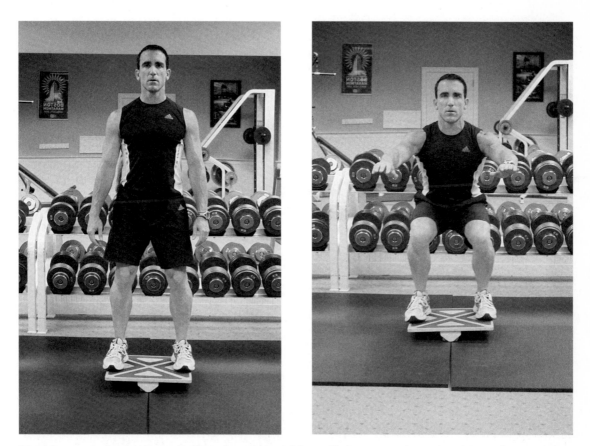

Stand on a balance board. Your feet should be a little more than shoulder-width apart with your toes pointing forward. Keeping your chest up and your knees behind your toes, lower your body to just above 90 degrees of knee bend, hold for 1 second, then return to the starting position.

Balance Disc Squat

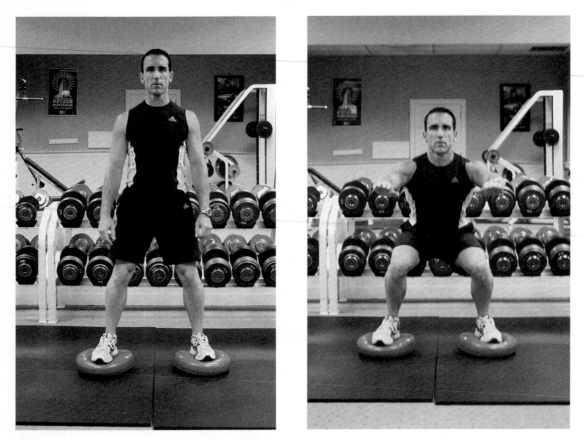

Stand with each foot on a balance disc. Your feet should be a little more than shoulder-width apart with your toes pointing forward. Keeping your chest up and your knees behind your toes, lower your body to just above 90 degrees of knee bend, hold for 1 second, then return to the starting position.

Single-Leg Ball Squat

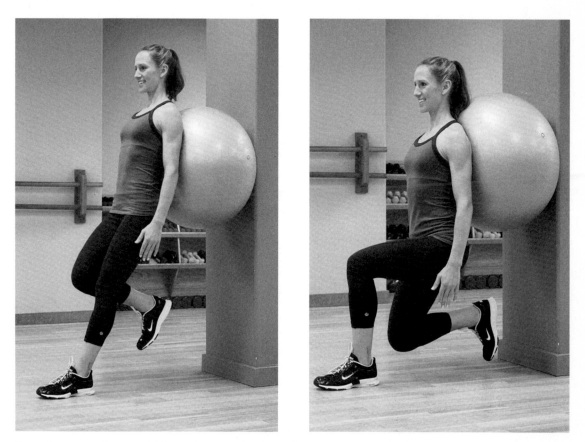

Stand on one leg, positioned towards the middle of your body, pressing a stability ball into a wall with your back. Keeping your chest up and your knee behind your toes, lower your body to just above 90 degrees of knee bend, hold for 1 second, then return to the starting position.

Bench Jump

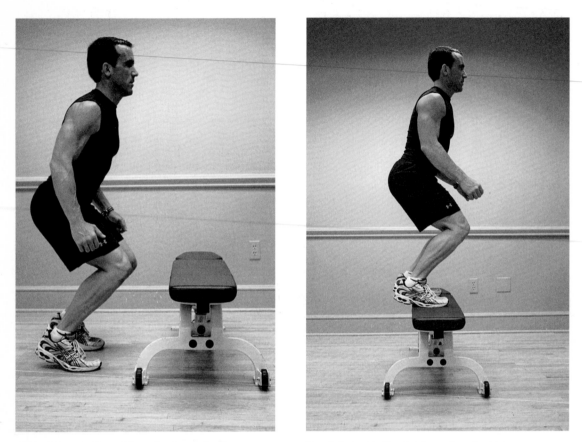

Standing at the side of a bench, jump up onto it with both feet, then back down, repeating as fast as possible.

Bench Split Jump

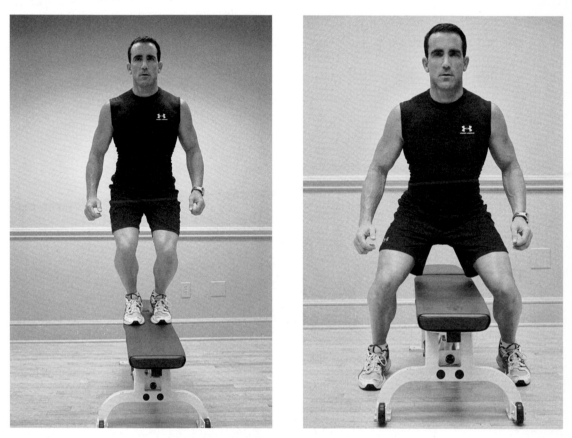

Standing on a bench, drop down to the floor with your feet on either side of the bench, then jump back up, repeating as fast as possible.

Trainer Tip: Do not make body-weight exercises too difficult too soon.

All too often I see someone doing a body-weight exercise with dumbbells when he or she shouldn't be. He or she is not yet good enough or strong enough at that movement to be adding resistance, and the exercise suffers as a result. It can also lead to injury, especially during exercises such as squats and lunges. Master the movement first. When you do add weight, be especially careful to keep strict form throughout.

Ask a Trainer: What does "BOSU" stand for?

BOSU is an acronym for "BOth Sides Up." A piece of exercise equipment that looks like a big ball cut in half, it is used to make exercises more unstable. The "BOth Sides Up" part refers to the fact that you can use it with either the flat side or the rounded side on the ground.

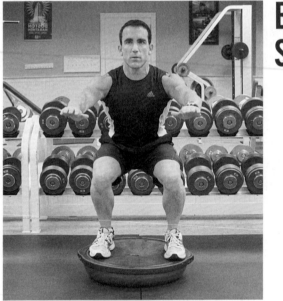

BOSU Squat

An unstable squat.

Cables

Though cables usually fall under the umbrella of selectorized machines, I feel they need their own category. Now also known as functional trainers, cables, like free weights, provide an infinite number of exercise possibilities.

Cable Rope Crunch

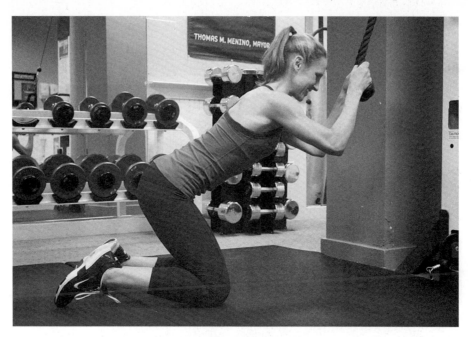

Kneeling on the floor while holding the rope attachment near your head, bend at the waist, bringing your elbows toward your knees. Pause for 1 second, then return to the starting position.

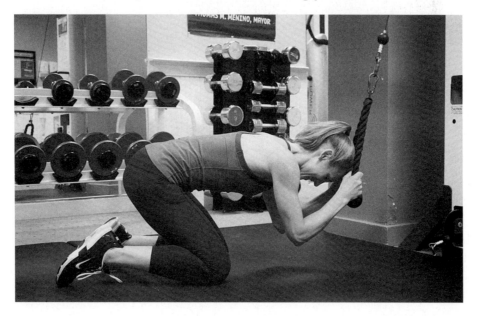

Cable Oblique Rope Crunch

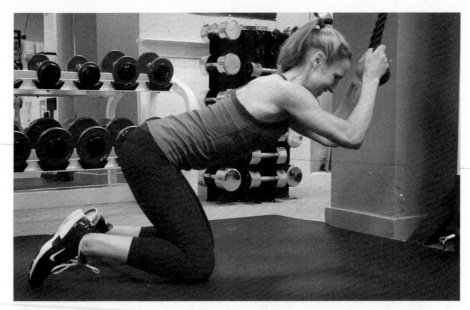

Kneeling on the floor while holding the rope attachment near your head, bend and twist at the waist, bringing your left elbow toward your right knee. Return to the starting position, then repeat to the other side.

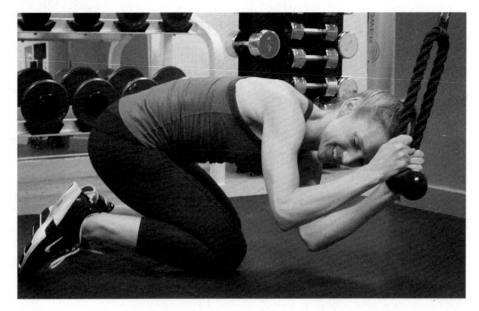

Cable Chest Press

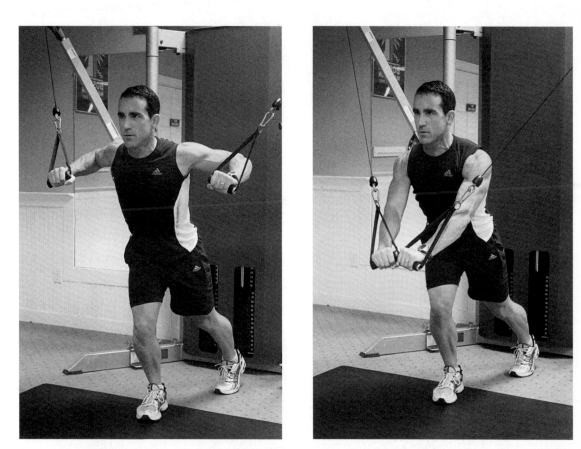

Stand holding a handle attachment in either hand with your palms facing down. Press your arms out in front of your chest until they are almost touching, then return to the starting position.

Cable Fly

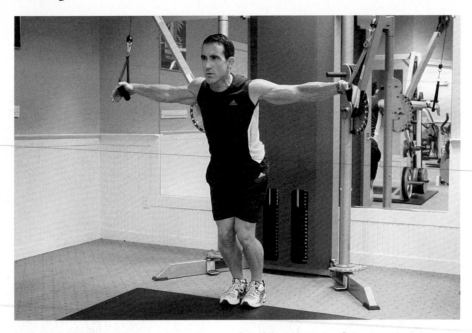

Stand holding a handle attachment in either hand with your palms facing forward. Bring them together in front of your chest and touch your palms together, then return to the starting position.

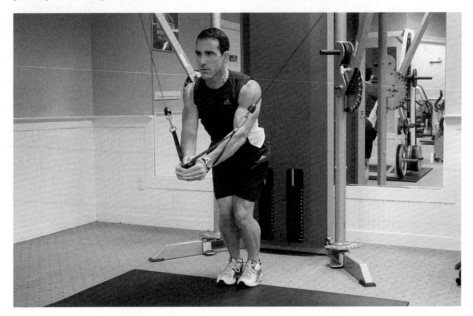

Cable Biceps Curl, Handle

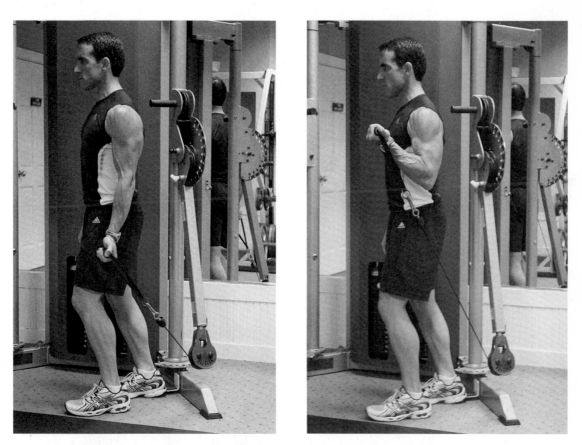

Stand holding the handle attachment at your side. Bending at the elbow, raise the handle toward your shoulder, hold for 1 second, then slowly lower it.

Cable Biceps Curl, Straight Bar

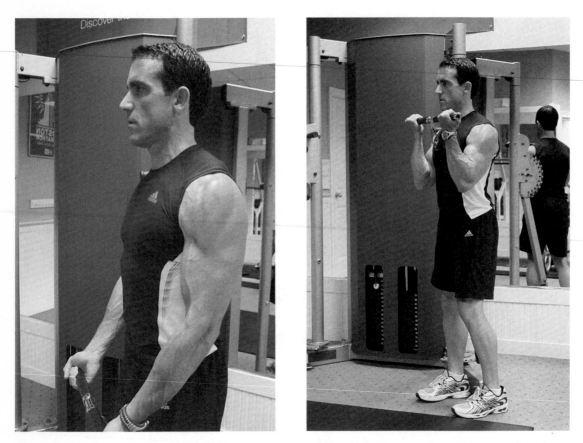

Stand holding the straight bar in front of your thighs. Bending at the elbows, raise the bar toward your shoulders, hold for 1 second, then slowly lower it.

Cable Shoulder Front Raise, Straight Bar

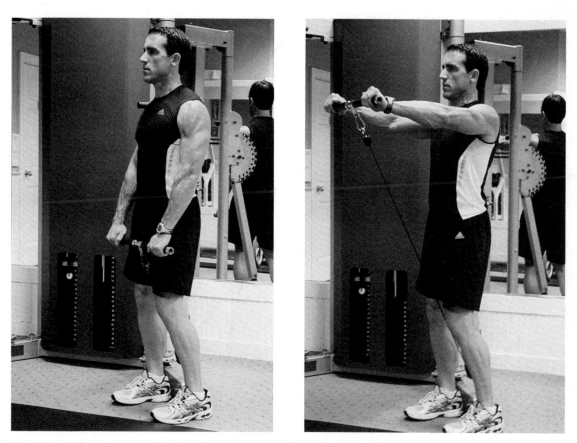

Stand holding the straight bar in front of your thighs with your back toward the cable machine and the cable between your legs. Keeping your elbows slightly bent, raise the bar to shoulder height, hold for 1 second, then slowly lower it.

Cable Shoulder Lateral Raise, Handle

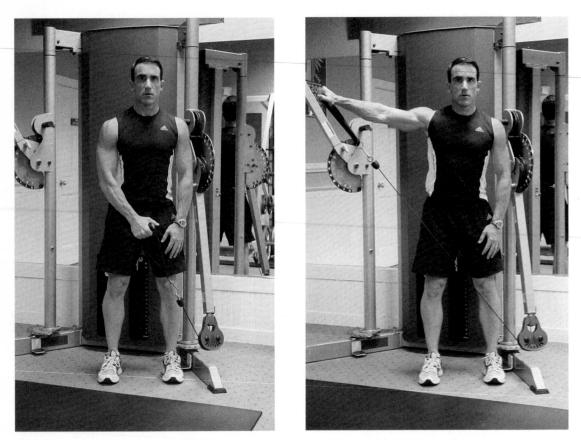

Stand holding the handle attachment at your side with your palm facing your body. With a slight bend in your elbow, raise the handle out to the side and up to shoulder height, hold for 1 second, then slowly lower it.

Cable Shoulder Front Raise, Handle

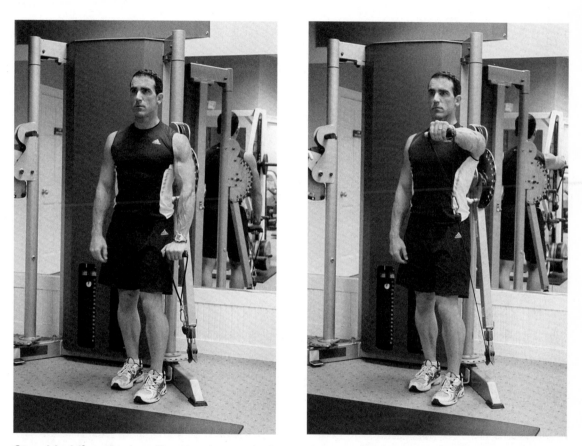

Stand holding the handle attachment in front of your thigh. With a slight bend in your elbow, raise the handle in front of you up to shoulder height, hold for 1 second, then slowly lower it.

Cable Shoulder Internal Rotation

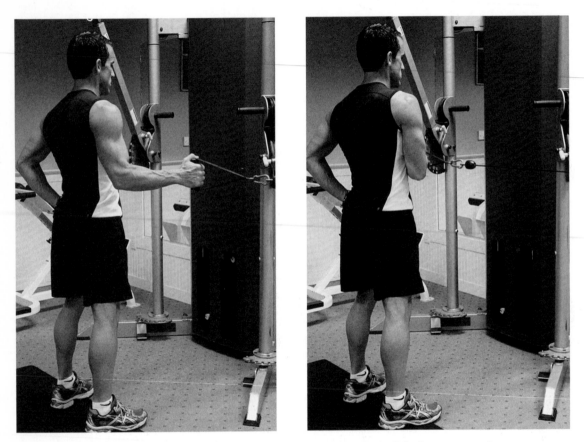

Stand holding the handle attachment with your arm bent to 90 degrees and your upper arm pressed against your body. Keeping your forearm parallel to the floor, pull the handle toward your body, hold for 1 second, then return to the starting position.

Cable Shoulder External Rotation

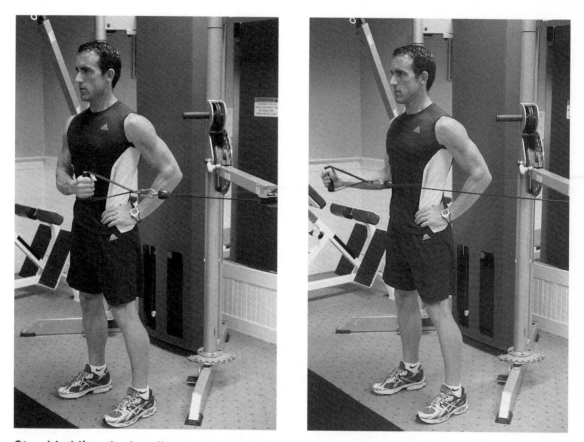

Stand holding the handle attachment with your arm bent to 90 degrees and your upper arm pressed against your body. Keeping your forearm parallel to the floor, pull the handle away from your body, hold for 1 second, then return to the starting position.

Cable Bent-Over Triceps Kickback, Handle

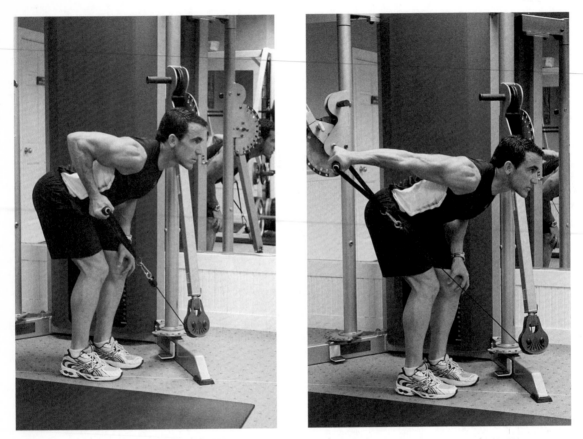

Stand facing the cable machine, holding a handle attachment with one hand, bent over at the waist, with your upper arm parallel to the floor and your palm facing forward. Pull the handle away from you until your arm is fully extended behind you, hold for 1 second, then return to the starting position.

Cable Triceps Extension, V-Bar

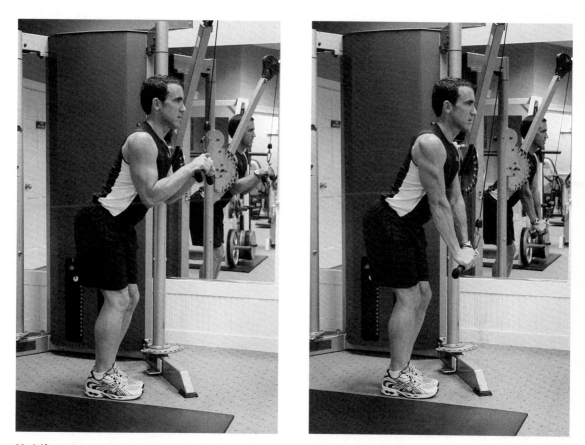

Holding the V-bar attachment, press the cable down toward the floor until your arms are fully extended, hold for 1 second, then slowly return to the starting position. Be sure to keep your elbows fixed throughout the entire movement.

Cable Triceps Extension, Rope

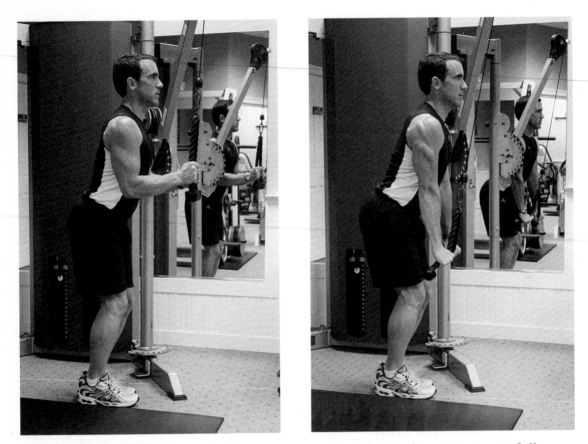

Holding the rope attachment, pull it down toward the floor until your arms are fully extended, hold for 1 second, then slowly return to the starting position. Be sure to keep your elbows fixed throughout the entire movement.

Cable Triceps Extension, Straight Bar, Prone Grip

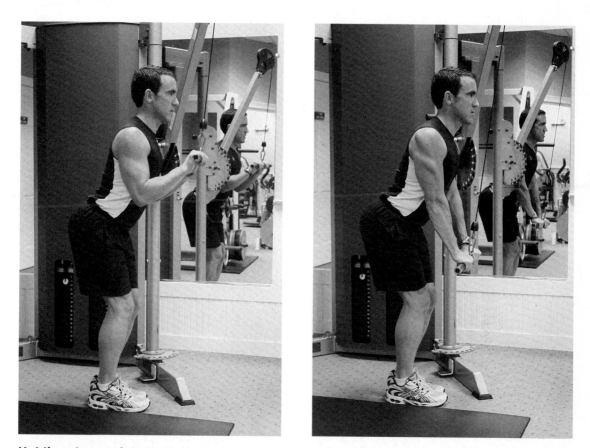

Holding the straight bar attachment with your palms facing down, press it down toward the floor until your arms are fully extended, hold for 1 second, then slowly return to the starting position. Be sure to keep your elbows fixed throughout the entire movement.

Cable Triceps Extension, Straight Bar, Supine Grip

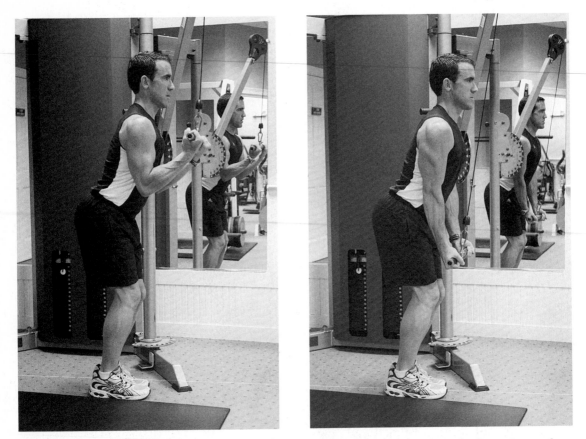

Holding the straight bar attachment with your palms facing up, press it down toward the floor until your arms are fully extended, hold for 1 second, then slowly return to the starting position. Be sure to keep your elbows fixed throughout the entire movement.

Cable Skull Crusher

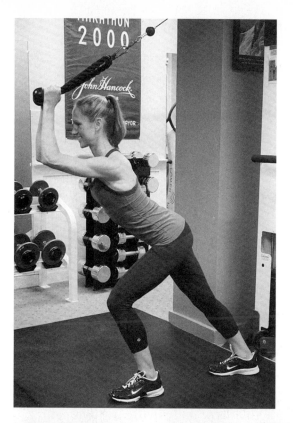

Stand with your back to the cable machine, holding the rope attachment over your head with your arms bent. Press the rope away from you until your arms are fully extended, hold for 1 second, then slowly return to the starting position.

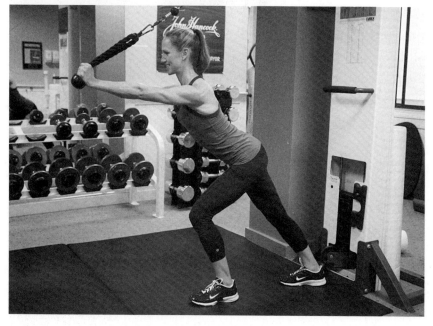

Ask a Trainer: Which is better? Free weights or machines?

Neither one is "better" per se. It depends. It depends on numerous factors, including your goals, age, fitness knowledge, and fitness level. The newer you are to working out, the more machines you should use at the beginning. The machines will allow you to build your strength gradually and safely. You can get started on them with just a brief orientation. You can do an easy strength circuit using machines. As you get stronger and more confident, you can gradually begin introducing free weights into your program.

Core Exercises

I know what you want, what you really want when it comes to working out. You want flat abs. Everyone does. And everyone can have them, yes, *everyone*, if they're willing to work for them. I don't care what your genetics are, or your metabolism, or your body type. If you do what you need to do, you can have the abs you've always wanted.

But it's not just about the abs. You also need to do lower back exercises. More than 80 percent of us will have lower back problems at some point in our lives. But we don't have to. A strong core (your abs, lower back, and glutes) is essential to being able to perform our activities of daily living without pain.

Realize also that abdominals are not just about looks; a weak abdominal wall is often one of the causes of lower back pain. How is that possible? you may ask. It's simple: the abdominals are in front of the lower back and part of the core. When the abs are weak, the strength of the core is compromised, and lower back pain is often the result. Strong abdominal muscles are not just about vanity.

A strong core is also essential to sports performance. I don't care what your level of proficiency is at your particular sport, core training will not only make you better, it will also protect you from potential injury.

While I could just focus on helping you get flat abs, I also want to help you avoid back pain. You can do both in minimal time if you work out intelligently.

Lower back exercises are boring. I get it. I don't enjoy doing them, either. They seem stupid. While you are doing them, they feel like a complete waste of time. Well, mark my words; I will repeat this phrase over and over because it is so important: either you will do these exercises now, or you will pay a physical therapist to make you do them after you have gotten injured. Many of you will recognize them because you have already done them in therapy. Well, do them. Just a few minutes a few times a week will make all the difference in the world.

Here are some of the most effective core exercises to sculpt your abs, improve your sports performance, and keep you injury-free. You can have it all.

Hanging Bent-Knee Raise

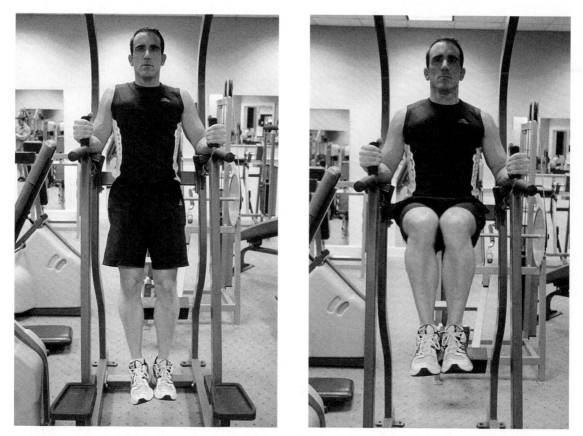

Holding your body up in a dip station or with straps, bend your knees to 90 degrees and pull them toward your chest, squeezing your abs, then slowly lower your knees to the starting position.

Hanging Oblique Raise

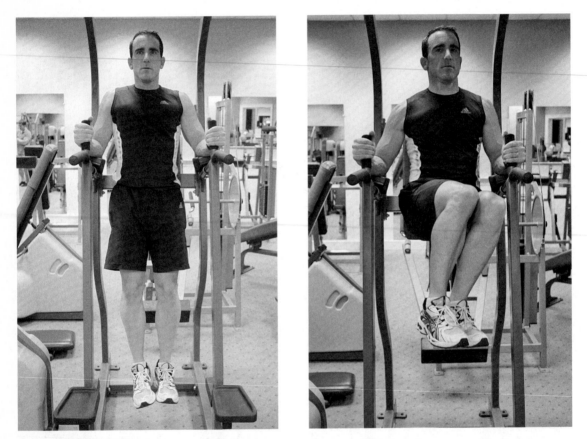

Holding your body up in a dip station or with straps, bend your knees to 90 degrees and then twist them up and to the right, squeezing your abs. Slowly lower your knees back to the starting position, then twist while pulling them up and to the left.

Hanging Straight-Knee Raise

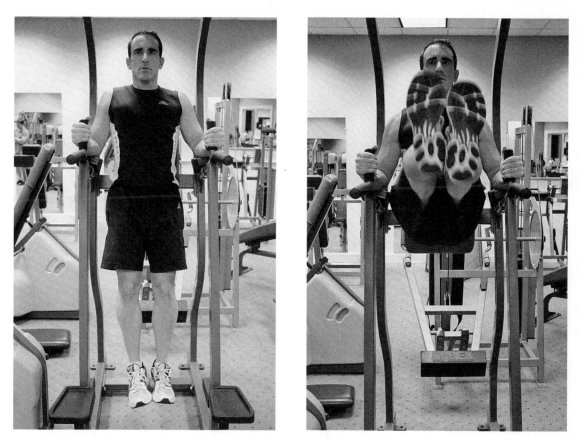

Holding your body up in a dip station or with straps with your legs straight, lift your legs as high as you can, hold for 1 second, then slowly lower them to the starting position.

Plank

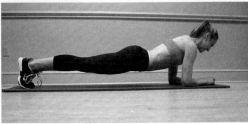

Assume a push-up position but support your upper body with your forearms and your palms pressed onto the floor. Keep your body perfectly straight and your abdominals pulled tight, yet breathing normally.

Side Plank

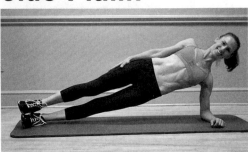

Lie on your side with one arm bent underneath you at 90 degrees and your opposite arm resting on your body. Raise your hips and legs off the ground until your body forms a straight line and hold.

Straight-Arm Plank

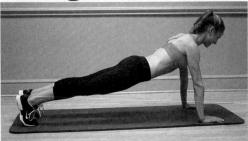

Assume the "up" push-up position, with your arms fully extended and your body perfectly straight. Keep your abdominals tight and hold.

Two-Point Side Plank

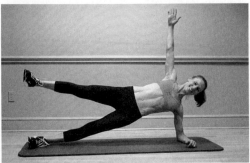

Lie on one side with your arm bent underneath you at 90 degrees and your opposite arm resting on your body. Raise your hips and legs off the ground until your body forms a straight line, then raise one arm and one leg and hold.

Alternating-Leg Plank

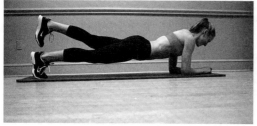

Assume a push-up position but support your upper body with your forearms and your palms pressed onto the floor. Keep your body perfectly straight and your abdominals pulled tight, yet breathing normally. Alternate raising and lowering a foot while maintaining your form.

Ball Plank

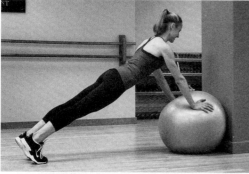

Assume the "up" push-up position on a stability ball, with your arms fully extended and your body perfectly straight. Keep your abdominals tight and hold.

Ball Plank with Raised Leg

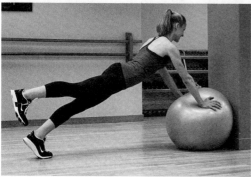

Assume the "up" push-up position on a stability ball, with your arms fully extended and your body perfectly straight. Keep your abdominals tight and hold. Alternate raising and lowering a foot while maintaining your form.

Ball Crunch

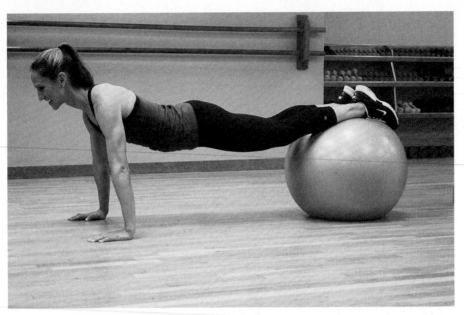

Assume the "up" push-up position but with your lower legs and the top of your feet on a stability ball. Pull the ball toward your body, hold for 1 second, then return to the starting position.

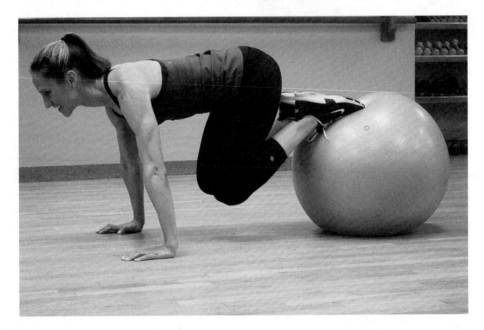

Crunch, Hands Across Chest

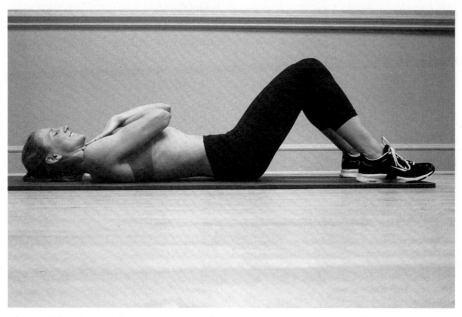

Lie on the floor with your knees bent and your hands folded across your chest. Keeping your chin off of your chest, slowly lift your upper body off the floor, hold for 1 second, then lower.

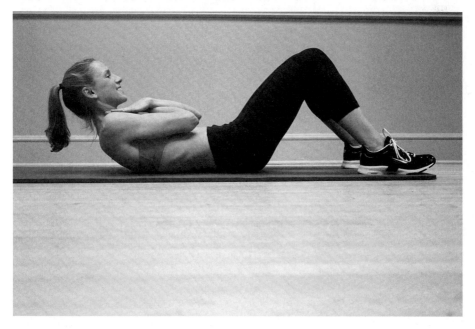

Oblique Crunch

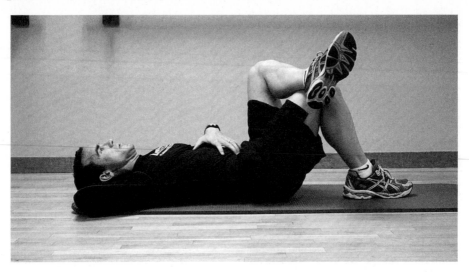

Lie on the floor with your right knee bent and your left leg crossed over, with the ankle resting on the thigh. Place your right hand behind your head, then bring that elbow toward your raised foot while twisting and bringing that shoulder blade up off the floor. Do the prescribed number of repetitions, then switch arms and legs and repeat to the other side.

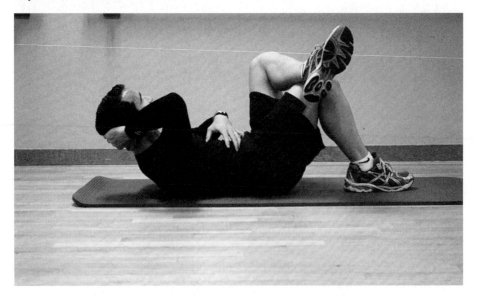

Side Crunch

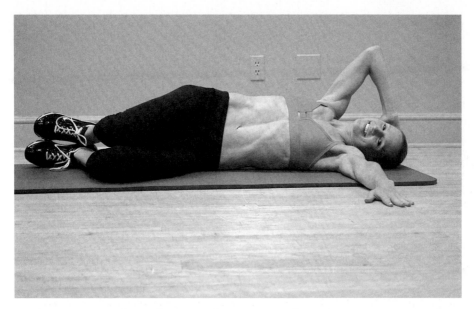

Lie on your left side with your right arm behind your head, your knees bent to 90 degrees, and your left arm on the floor in front of you for balance. Bring your elbow toward your hip, hold for 1 second, then lower and repeat.

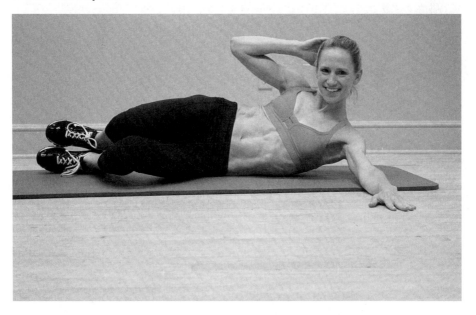

Side Crunch with Raised Leg

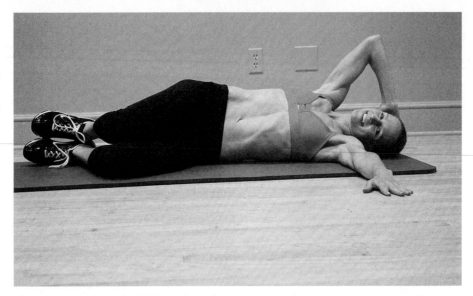

Lie on your left side with your right arm behind your head, your knees bent to 90 degrees, and your left arm on the floor in front of you for balance. Bring your elbow toward your hip as you lift your legs off the ground, hold for 1 second, then lower your legs and repeat.

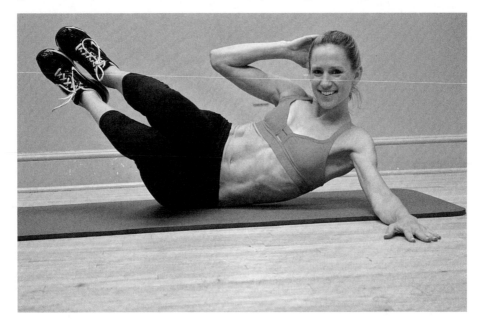

Double Crunch

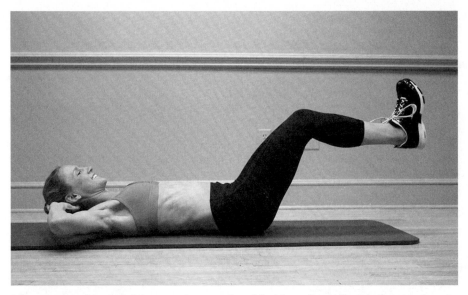

Lie on your back with your legs raised in the air and your knees bent to 90 degrees. Making sure to keep your lower back pressed to the floor (a reverse pelvic tilt), bring your chest up toward your knees, then lower back down to the starting position.

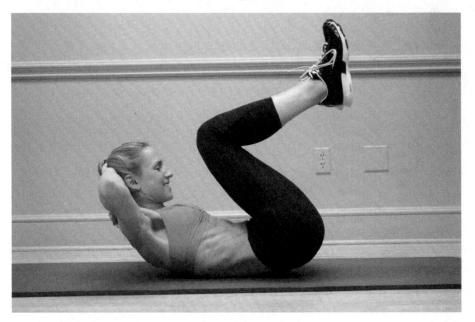

Bench Crunch

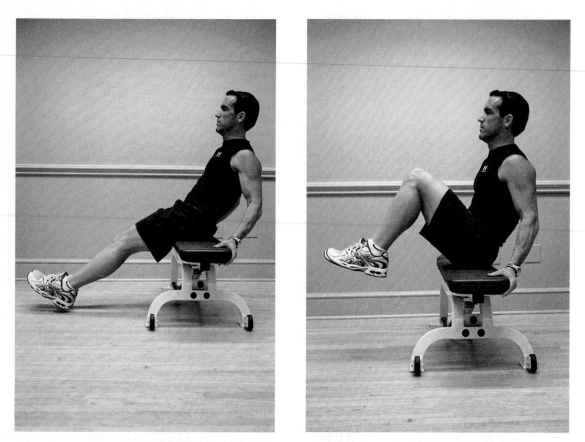

Sit on a bench, leaning slightly back with your legs raised and bent to 90 degrees. Pull your knees toward your chest, hold for 1 second, then return to the starting position.

Bicycle Crunch

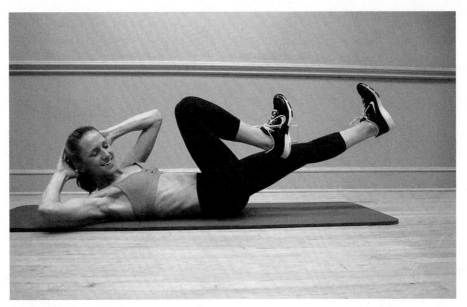

Lying on your back with your hands behind your head, alternate bringing your right elbow to your left knee and your left elbow to your right knee. Keep your abdominals tight throughout.

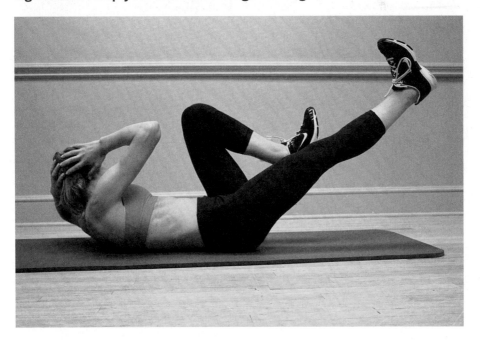

Seal

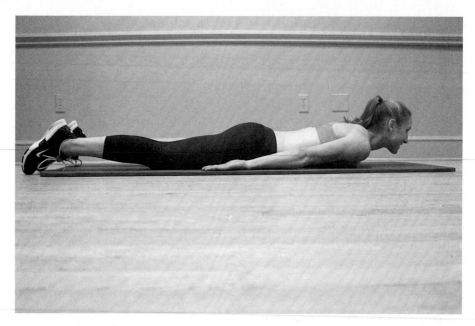

Lie on the floor with your hands at your sides. Simultaneously lift your upper body and your feet up off the floor, squeezing the muscles of your lower back. Hold for 1 second, then slowly lower.

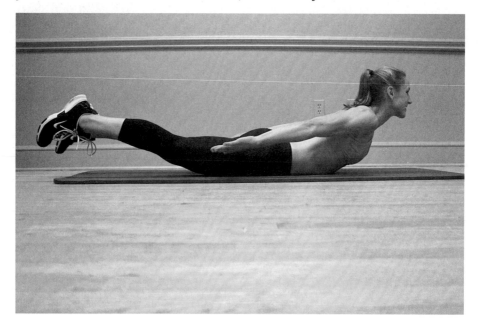

Bird Dog

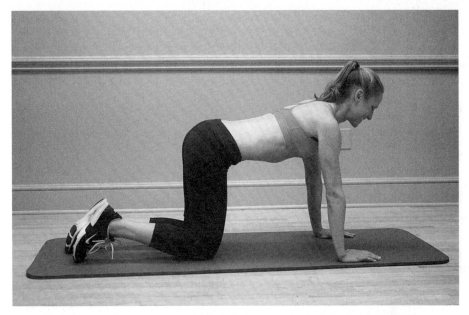

Kneeling on all fours, extend your left arm and right leg, hold for 1 second, and return to the starting position. Then extend your right arm and left leg, hold for 1 second, and return to the starting position.

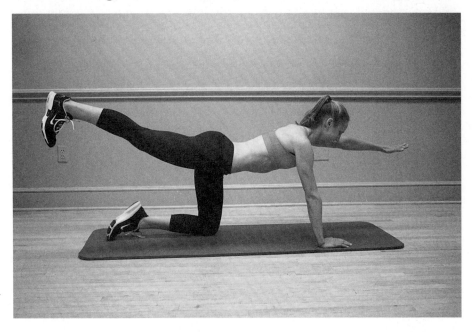

Two-Point Plank

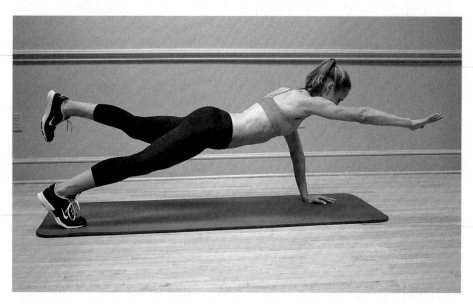

Hold your body in the "up" push-up position. Raise your right arm and left leg, hold for 1 second, and return to the starting position. Then raise your left arm and right leg, hold for 1 second, and return to the starting position.

Superman

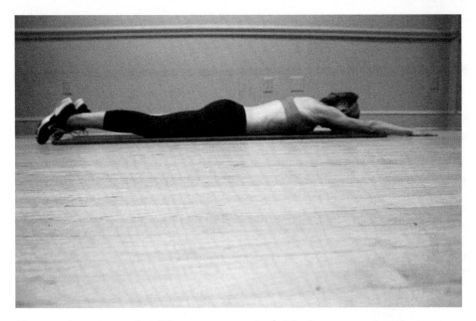

Lie on your stomach with your arms straight above your head. Simultaneously lift both hands and feet up off the floor, squeezing the muscles of your lower back. Hold for 1 second, then slowly lower.

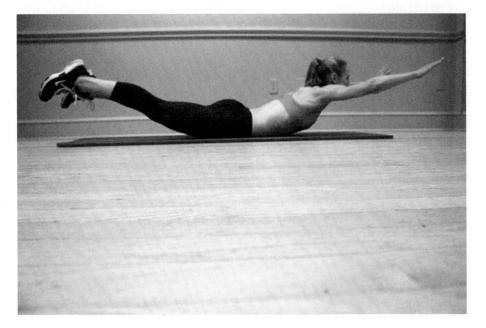

Rule 1: Men Lift Weights That Are Too Heavy, Women Lift Weights That Are Too Light

Men think they are Arnold, and women are afraid of becoming Arnold. Both couldn't be further from the truth. This may sound like an oversimplification, but trust me, it's not. It's one of the primary reasons people do not see results from their strength training. With men the major problem is ego: they want to impress the other guys in the gym. You can bench-press 250 pounds? Watch me do 275. It's crazy to me. I couldn't care less about being stronger than a bunch of other guys at the gym. Who cares? It only leads to bad form, decreased results, and inevitable injury. My goal is to do the most effective workout I can possibly do. I want to look great in the twenty-three hours I'm outside the gym, not impress a bunch of guys I don't even know for the hour I'm working out.

And women's problem? It's the "B" word that makes my skin crawl.

Bulky.

Women are petrified of getting bulky. They have been led to believe that if they lift even moderately heavy weights, they will get arms like Arnold and legs like tree trunks. This couldn't be further from the truth. They focus instead on working out with low weights and high repetitions, using weights that are significantly lighter than objects they lift all day long, such as a gallon of milk or their children. What they end up doing is working the endurance capabilities of the muscles without making any meaningful changes whatsoever. It's a waste of time.

Trainer Tip: Find a workout partner.

Let's face it, working out by yourself can be pretty difficult. I highly recommend finding a workout partner to maximize your program. A workout buddy is a great idea for numerous reasons. He or she can:

1. **PROVIDE MOTIVATION.** The days you don't want to work out, she will get you out the door. The days she feels like skipping, you will get her to the gym. When you want to give up completely, she will talk you into sticking with your plan.

2. **SERVE AS SPOTTERS.** Especially when you are doing the bench press or squats, your partner can help spot you, keeping your workouts safer yet challenging at the same time.

3. **INCREASE YOUR EXERCISE ARSENAL.** There are numerous strength moves you can do with your partner, such as crunches with a medicine ball and partner push-ups. These are fun and very effective.

4. **PROVIDE COMPANIONSHIP.** Working out can be lonely, especially during long cardio sessions. Having a friend next to you to talk with while you slave away on the elliptical trainer can make the time fly by.

5. **PROVIDE COMPETITION.** Let's be honest, as human beings we like to compete with one another. I recommend finding a workout partner who is just a little fitter, just a little stronger than you are. By trying to keep up with that person, you will challenge yourself in ways that you cannot do alone.

Don't have a workout partner? Start looking around the gym during your workouts. Chances are there is someone who trains alone at the same time you do, and he or she may be in the market for a partner as well. Look for someone who seems to have similar goals. Start gradually by striking up casual conversations with that person. Have him or her spot you for a few exercises. After you have gotten to know each other a little bit, invite him or her to do a workout with you. Get on the StairMaster and work out side by side. Once you feel you know him or her well enough, ask if he or she wants to meet you at the gym on certain days so you can help each other reach your goals.

It doesn't have to be just one person, either. Many gyms have small groups of people who meet regularly and exercise together. There is incredible power in numbers. Consider creating your own workout group; the more people, the better. A small group takes away the awkwardness that can exist in the one-on-one dynamic. And if one person doesn't show up, no problem; you have several other people to work out with.

Consider asking at the front desk or the trainer's office if they could recommend someone for you to work out with. A gym employee can help. You might even be paired up with someone with whom you could become interested in splitting personal training sessions. Doing semiprivate sessions will save you money while giving you two people to be accountable to. Just remember that if you do pay to train with a partner, make sure he or she is as fit as or a little fitter than you. If not, you may be shortchanged during the workout.

Trainer Tip: Do cardio workouts with a partner.

One fun way to do your cardio workout with a partner is as follows: Get onto cardio equipment side by side. It doesn't matter what kind: the Gauntlet, treadmill, rowing machine, whatever. Start with a warm-up of five minutes or so, then alternate calling out intervals. Let's say you are both running on a treadmill. You may say, "Two minutes at 7.0 miles per hour"; then you both run at that pace. Then she may say, "Sixty-second second hill at an incline of 6.0," and you will do that. Continue to alternate coaching each other for the duration of the workout. It's a really fun way to mix up your routine.

Fit Myth: You can "lengthen" a muscle.

Nope. This is the never-ending pitch of so many fitness products and workout routines that are playing into the whole "bulk" myth. Let's put it this way: Your muscles have what is known as an "origin" and an "insertion." Both are fixed and attached to bones. In order to "lengthen" a muscle, therefore, you'd have to detach the muscle and reattach it farther down the bone.

You have genetically predetermined muscle characteristics. You are an ectomorph, mesomorph, or endomorph, meaning that you have a skinny frame, muscular frame, or big frame, respectively. Focused strength training will give you the best body you are genetically capable of achieving. An endomorph can never become an ectomorph, but that doesn't mean that the endomorph cannot have a great body. You want to do total-body workouts, targeting all of the major muscles, regardless of which of the three body types you possess.

Breaking Down the Body

As you strength train, I want you to constantly think of the body in terms of the following "regions." Make sure to work all of them, not just the ones you want to change. You don't always need to do full body workouts like during circuit training sessions, but remember that you cannot spot reduce. And yes, guys, you do have to work your legs as well.

UPPER BODY

1. Chest
2. Back
3. Shoulders

4. Biceps

5. Triceps

LOWER BODY

1. Glutes (butt)

2. Quads (front of thighs)

3. Hamstrings (back of upper legs)

4. Calves

ABS

1. Rectus abdominis (front of abs—the "six-pack")

2. Obliques (side of abs)

3. Lower Abs (below the belly button)

LOWER BACK

1. Spinal Erectors (lower back)

Whenever you exercise, you want to focus on these muscle groups. So if you were doing an upper-body day, you would focus on the five major muscle groups of chest, back, shoulders, biceps, and triceps. On your leg days you want to target the four areas of the butt, quads, hamstrings, and calves. For abs? Break it down into three sections: front, side, and lower. Lower back is pretty much just lower back.

Lifting Lingo: Compound Exercise

Compound exercises are multijoint exercises that work several muscles at one time. Since they work multiple muscle groups simultaneously, doing these exercises is a great way to shorten your workout time. The squat and the bench press are examples of compound exercises. Biceps curls and triceps kickbacks are known as "isolation exercises," as they work only one muscle at a time.

Rule 2: Do as Many Compound Exercises as Possible to Maximize Your Results

OTHER BENEFITS OF DOING COMPOUND EXERCISES

1. They are more functional.

2. They can help improve balance and coordination.

3. They help improve sports performance.

4. They can burn more calories.

5. They can be combined with isolation exercises for the fastest possible workout.

OTHER COMPOUND EXERCISES

1. Leg press

2. Back row

3. Pull-up

4. Chin-up

5. Lunge

6. Shoulder press

7. Deadlift

8. Dip

Lifting Lingo: "Isometric" versus "isotonic"

Most of the exercises we think of as strength training are known as *isotonic* exercises. They involve both a lengthening and shortening of a muscle, such as the biceps during a biceps curl. The lengthening happens as you lower the weight, and the shortening occurs when you raise it. An *isometric* exercise also strengthens the muscle, but without lengthening or shortening it. Confused? An easy example would be a plank. There is no movement, no lengthening or shortening of a muscle, yet you gain strength by doing such exercises. Disciplines such as yoga and Pilates often involve isometric exercises.

QUICK FACTS ABOUT ISOMETRIC EXERCISES

1. They are not truly "functional" exercises. Holding a certain pose for an extended period of time does make you stronger, but not in a real-world functional way.

2. They give you strength at the specific angle at which you exercise. Research has shown that isometric exercises make you strong at the angle at the which you perform them. So if you push against a wall and hold it, you will get stronger at doing that particular movement. This would be most beneficial to someone like a football lineman, whose sport requires him to be strong in this position.

3. They don't tone you the way isotonic exercises do. Please don't misunderstand me: there is a place for isometric exercises in almost everyone's exercise routine. When it comes to sculpting muscles, however, we need to overload them effectively through their full range of motion.

Exercise "Tweaks" to Make Exercises More Effective

It's not whether you do certain exercises that's important, it's whether or not you do them correctly.

1. **DUMBBELL FLYES**

    MISTAKE: Using a weight that is too heavy

    Most people do chest flyes incorrectly, using weight that is too heavy, so that the movement ends up becoming a modified chest press instead of a true chest fly.

    FIX: Go lighter. Let your ego go. Use an amount of weight that you can control, keeping it as far away from your body as possible while maintaining just a slight bend in your elbow. The heavier the weight, the harder it is to hold out from your body. In order to make this exercise different from the chest press, you have to use a lighter, more manageable weight.

Dumbbell Chest Fly—Bad

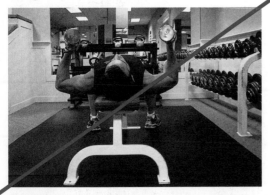

The weights are too close to the body. This is a cross between a chest press and a fly, and not a good version of either.

Dumbbell Chest Fly—Good

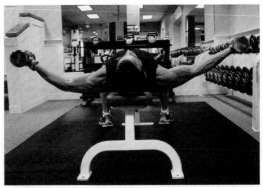

The weights are light and manageable. They can be held open and away from the body.

2. SINGLE-ARM DUMBBELL BENT-OVER ROWS

MISTAKE: Keeping a rounded upper back

Back exercises in general, and rows in particular, are so often done incorrectly, with a rounded back being one of the most common mistakes. When your back is rounded, it turns this exercise into an arm exercise instead of one targeting the back; it works the biceps a little and the lats not at all.

FIX: Pull your shoulders back.

You want to drop your shoulders and keep them pulled back. I start clients off by having them stand with perfect posture. They then bend slowly at the waist, maintaining this posture throughout the entire exercise. A trainer will often place his fingers on a client's shoulder blades to get him to initiate the movement from the back instead of the arms.

Dumbbell Row—Good

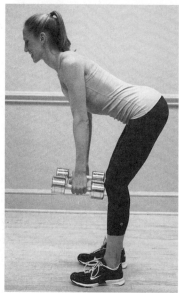

Dumbbell Row—Bad

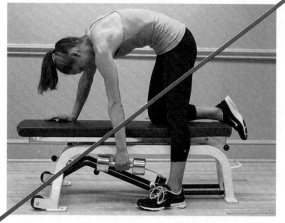

The back is rounded. This becomes an arm exercise with little to no back involvement.

The back is flat, with the natural lordotic curve. The neck is relaxed.

3. BICEPS CURL

MISTAKE: Moving the elbow

So much of the effectiveness of the biceps curl lies in keeping the upper arm fixed. When the elbow moves, it takes the tension off of the biceps and lessens the positive stress on the muscle.

FIX: Keep your elbow fixed in space.

Whether you're using a dumbbell, barbell, cable attachment, whatever; when doing a biceps curl, make sure that your elbow does not move at all. If you have major problems keeping your elbow from moving, try lightening the weight. An inability to control the weight and to have to use momentum instead is often due to using a weight that is too heavy.

Dumbbell Biceps Curl—Bad

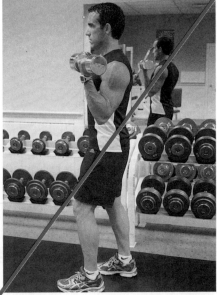

The elbow moves significantly during the exercise, taking the tension off of the muscle and allowing momentum to be used, significantly lessening the effectiveness of the exercise.

Dumbbell Biceps Curl—Good

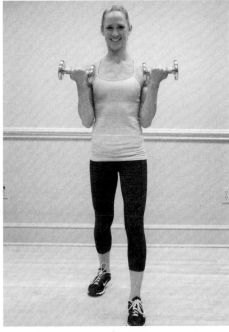

The elbow is close to the body and fixed in space. It doesn't move.

Ask a Trainer: How often can I do strength workouts? Can I do the same routine every day?

When you lift weights, you break down the muscle fibers you are working. These fibers need time to rebuild themselves, a minimum of one day. So you do not want to work the same muscle group two days in a row.

Ask a Trainer: But I want to lift weights six days a week, with one day off to rest completely. How can I do this?

Here are a few ways in which you can structure your weekly strength training routine:

WEEK NO.	MONDAY	TUESDAY	WEDNESDAY	THURSDAY	FRIDAY	SATURDAY	SUNDAY
1	Upper body	Lower body	Upper body	Lower body	Upper body	Lower body	REST
2	Full body	REST	Full body	REST	Full body	REST	REST
3	Chest, shoulders, triceps	Back, biceps	Legs	Chest, shoulders, triceps	Back, biceps	Legs	REST
4	Chest, back	Shoulders, biceps, triceps	Legs	Chest, back	Shoulders, biceps, triceps	Legs	REST
5	Legs	Chest, shoulders, triceps	Back, biceps	Legs	Chest, shoulders, triceps	Back, biceps	REST

Trainer Tip: Make Monday your legs day.

Guys love to bench-press, and they love to do it on Mondays. Chances are good that if you schedule your chest workout for Monday, you will have to wait for benches, dumbbells, and chest machines. The smartest way to schedule your routine is to do legs on Monday. Trust me, you'll have the leg press and squat rack all to yourself.

Rule 3: Do These Three Exercises Now, or You'll Pay a Physical Therapist to Make You Do Them Later

1. **LEG EXTENSIONS.** Bad knees? Many knee problems are due to an unstable knee joint, often caused by muscle weakness in general and weakness of the vastus medialis oblique muscle in particular. Referred to as the "VMO" by physical therapists, the vastus medialis oblique can be targeted and strengthened by doing leg extensions.

Machine Leg Extension

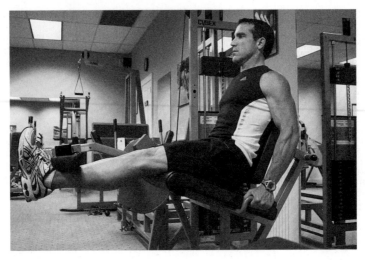

Either do these now or in therapy.

2. **BACK EXTENSIONS.** More than 80 percent of people will have back pain at some point in their lives. Our sedentary lives are making our backs weaker and weaker. The good news is that just a few sets of back extensions done a few times a week is all you need to strengthen and protect your lower back.

Back Extension

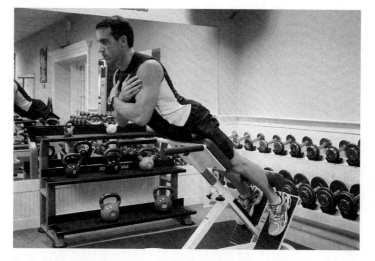

These will save you lots of money in physical therapy bills as well.

3. **INTERNAL/EXTERNAL SHOULDER ROTATION.** Anyone who has experienced a shoulder injury and had to do rehab for it knows exactly what these exercises are. Usually done with a light dumbbell, cable, or rubber tubing, these two exercises involves keeping your upper arm pressed against your side while rotating your arm away from your body and toward it while bent at a right angle. These are really painful when you do them right after rotator cuff surgery (I had my right shoulder done in high school after a football injury). If you do them while you are healthy, they may be boring, but they can potentially prevent major shoulder issues. Do a few sets during your workout to strengthen the shoulder joint and avoid having to do them in a physical therapist's office.

Cable Internal Shoulder Rotation

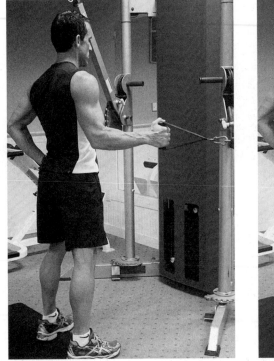

This exercise works wonders.

Ask a Trainer: What is the rotator cuff?

The rotator cuff consists of four muscles: the supraspinatus, the infraspinatus, teres minor, and subscapularis. These muscles work together to stabilize the shoulder joint. Chances are good that if you have shoulder pain, one or more of these muscles is to blame.

Cable External Shoulder Rotation

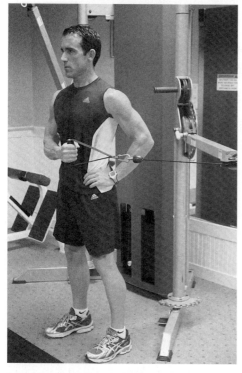 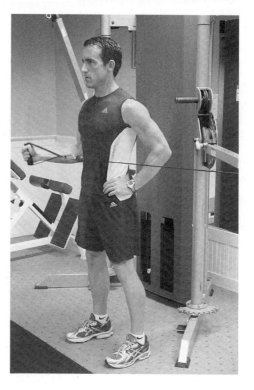

Strengthening and protecting your shoulders.

Rule 4: You Can't Spot Reduce Fat from Your Body

This is one of the top workout mistakes. It results in so much wasted time and effort. What exactly is "spot reduction"? It's when you work a specific area in the hopes of slimming it down.

Unfortunately, the body does not work that way.

You cannot tell your body where to decrease its fat stores by simply targeting a particular area with exercise. We all have genetically predetermined areas where we store our fat. We also have genetically predetermined patterns that determine when and where we lose this fat. Here are the two biggest mistakes when it comes to spot reduction:

WOMEN: Hip abduction exercises. In an effort to trim down their hips, women will do any exercise that involves pushing the legs away from the body against resistance. Doesn't work.

MEN: Abs, abs, abs. Men waste an enormous amount of time trying to flatten ttheir guts through endless ab exercises. Say it with me now: abdominal exercises do not flatten; they strengthen. And when the excess fat around the middle is gone, ab exercises sculpt. But doing crunch after crunch when you have a spare tire around the middle will never get rid of that tire. Never.

So please do not fall for the spot reduction myth. I understand how confusing this concept is because we are bombarded with these very messages daily. The whole television fitness infomercial business is built around perpetuating this myth. It seems as though every week a new infomercial comes out that is trying to pitch yet another "flatten-those-abs" gizmo. Remember the ThighMaster? That created a whole generation of women with really strong thighs, not skinny ones.

Ask a Trainer: Is "locking out your knees" really bad for you during certain exercises?

No. You often hear that it's bad to lock out your knees during exercises such as the leg press and leg extension. Though you do want to avoid hyperextending, or taking the joint past extension, fully extending the leg to its natural endpoint is fine.

Machine Leg Extension

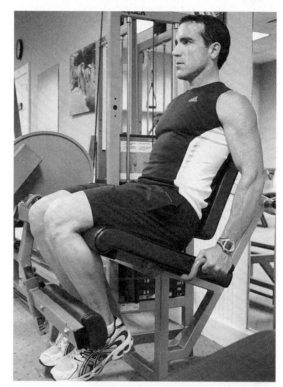

Raise the
weight, pause,
then lower it.

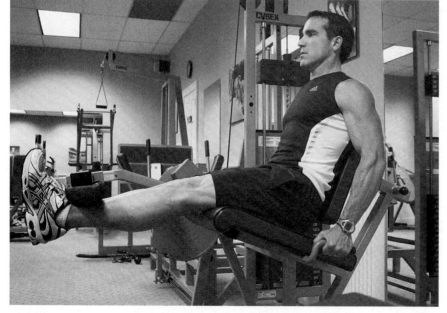

1. **CHANGE THE ORDER OF YOUR EXERCISES.** You can do the exact same exercises that you have always done. Just change the order in which you do them, and you will effectively change your routine.

2. **CHANGE YOUR GRIP.** By subtly changing your grip, you will significantly change an exercise. This can mean moving your hands closer or farther away on a barbell, using a palms-up instead of palms-down grip on a machine back row, or using a false grip on a dumbbell chest press.

Lifting Lingo: False Grip

A false grip refers to your thumb position while lifting weights. It means that instead of having your thumb underneath whatever you are gripping, you place it above. It doesn't matter if you are using dumbbells, a barbell, a kettlebell, or a machine; you can use a false grip with any of them. Why would you do this? I do not know of any studies that have looked at the muscle activation patterns of using this technique, but I do know through experience that certain exercises feel much more comfortable and even more effective when I use a false grip. To me, the subtle change feels as though it makes a big difference. Call it psychological, physical, or a combination of the two, it just feels as though I get a better contraction when using a false grip with certain exercises. Try it out and see how it feels.

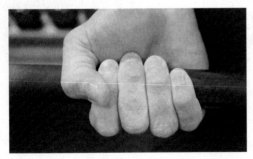

Regular Grip

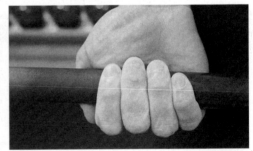

False Grip

3. **CHANGE THE ATTACHMENT.** When using equipment such as cables, you have a wide variety of attachments to choose from. Take a triceps exercise, for example. When using a cable to work this muscle, numerous options are available, including the rope attachment, V-bar, straight bar, stirrup handle, just the cable itself, and more. Change the attachment, and you will change the exercise.

4. **CHANGE THE TYPE OF WEIGHT.** If you are using free weights, switch to machines. If you are using machines, switch to cables. If you are using cables, change to body-weight exercises. Do the new routine for several weeks, then change it again.

5. **CHANGE YOUR GYM.** Just for a day. Every so often I go to a new gym and pay for a day pass. The change of scenery and the different equipment, surroundings, and people give a boost to my routine and revitalize my program.

Rule 5: Don't Do These Moves Anymore

I can't spend five minutes in a gym without wanting to go up to ten people and tell them what they are doing wrong and how to do it better. Here are a few of the most common errors I see on a daily basis.

1. **SIDE BENDS.** This abdominal, more specifically oblique, exercise is most commonly done while standing and holding a pair of dumbbells at your sides. You lower one dumbbell toward the floor, then the other, and continue alternating. This is an ineffective and unnatural movement. Your side abdominal muscles run on diagonal angles. To effectively train them, you want to perform a twisting motion, not a side bend. An example of a great exercise to do instead of side bends is the bicycle crunch.

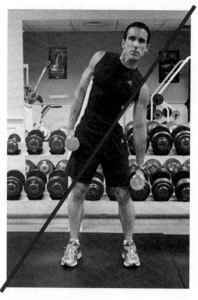

Side Bends

Please stop doing this.

2. **FULL SIT-UPS.** The days of the full sit-up are over. We "crunch" now. To do a true full sit-up requires an extraordinary amount of strength, which few people possess. In trying to do a full, old-school sit-up, people end up using a ridiculous amount of momentum, throwing their bodies around in order to raise their upper bodies completely off the floor. They often anchor their feet under something as well, significantly lessening the effectiveness of the exercise by bringing in the hip flexor muscles. Stop it. Focus on a much smaller range of motion, engaging only the abdominals as you lift your shoulder blades a few inches off the ground. This is more effective than the old-school crunch, and you won't throw out your neck or back in the process.

Full Sit-ups

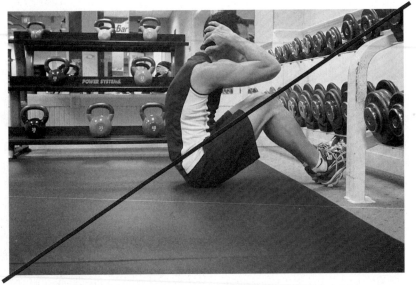

You don't need to go all the way up anymore.

3. **FAST BICEPS CURLS.** When doing alternating biceps curls with a dumbbell, wait until you complete one repetition before starting the next. Pumping and swinging the weights in rapid succession is not the way to go. Slow the movement down. Keep the tension on the muscles throughout the entire movement.

Rule 6: Don't Make an Exercise Too Hard

A great example of this is the walking lunge. I see so many people holding way too much weight while doing this exercise. They end up lunging down only an inch or two in order to control the weight, making the lunge almost worthless. Again, I'm all for working out hard, as you should now realize, but there is hard and then there is too hard.

Ask a Trainer: How many repetitions should I do?

GOAL	REPETITIONS
POWER	1–4
STRENGTH	4–8
TONING	10–15

Ask a Trainer: How many sets should I do?

One is good, two is better, and three is best when it come to muscle toning. To be honest, however, as I get older, I now have a difficult time doing three sets. I get too bored doing three sets of everything. I do two, but I make sure those two are incredibly effective. Use challenging weights, and really concentrate on your form.

If you are a power lifter, you will use heavy weights and do low repetitions, anywhere from one to four. If your primary goal is to build strength, you will also use heavier weights and shoot for anywhere from 4 to 8 repetitions. If you want to sculpt your body, you should do 10 to 15 reps with a manageable weight.

If you can easily do more than 15 repetitions, the weight is too light.

Trainer Tip: Use a weight for which the last few repetitions are difficult yet you can maintain proper form. When the final reps become easy, it is time to increase the weight.

Rule 7: Devote 10 Percent of Your Workout Session to Abs

As with my rule regarding cardio that you should do the same number of minutes per week as pounds you weigh, I have a rule when it comes to ab exercises: you should devote 10 percent of your workout session to abdominal exercises. So if you go to the gym for an hour, you should do six minutes worth of crunch-type exercises. Working out for thirty minutes? Do three minutes of ab exercises.

This ensures that you will make the most of your workout time. You need to focus first and foremost on burning calories and doing quality strength training. Ab exercises are a distant third when it comes to how much time at the gym should be devoted to them. Any extra time spent crunching away in vain is time that could be better spent elsewhere.

Rule 8: Don't Use the Floor and the Wall at the Gym. Use the Equipment!

You are paying good money for the equipment at the gym. You travel to get there. Then why would you spend the majority of your time doing crunches on the floor or stretching against a wall? Use as much of the equipment as you can! For example: instead of doing a traditional crunch while at the gym, use the hanging leg raise machine, do a rope crunch, or tighten your abs using a medicine ball or stability ball! You can do all of the other stuff at home. Or when you travel. Remember that one of the keys to fitness success is challenging your body in new ways. Frequently. By using as much of the equipment at the gym as possible to perform movements that your body is unaccustomed to doing, you will be well on your way to sculpting that perfect body.

Ask a Trainer: What is a body bar?

A body bar is a long, one-piece solid steel weighted fitness bar encased in rubber. Body bars come in a wide variety of weights and can be used for an infinite number of exercises. Preferred by women due to their lighter weight, they are often used in class settings such as total body conditioning classes. I personally use them for certain abdominal exercises, to work my shoulders, and even to help strengthen my shins. Be creative with them and add them to your routine.

Rule 9: The Top Three Exercises to Leave out of Your Routine

Not all exercises are created equal. Some have a much higher risk of injury than others. If these exercises were amazing and had the potential to radically change your body for the better, I would have a much different attitude toward them. But they don't. These three exercises can actually hurt you. The risk far outweighs the potential reward. I would therefore leave them out of your workout routine, no matter what your fitness level or goals.

1. **LYING STRAIGHT-LEG LIFTS.** Often referred to as the "six inches drill," this is an abdominal exercise where you lie on your back with your arms at your sides and your legs straight out in front of you. You then lift your legs a few inches off the ground and hold. Sometimes you raise them slightly higher and then lower them; another modification is to alternate opening and closing them while keeping them just off the floor.

Straight-Leg Lifts

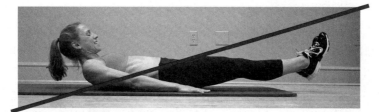

This move can really strain the lower back.

WHY IT'S BAD: This movement places an enormous amount of strain on the lower back. That's why some people stuff their hands underneath their butts for support while performing the move in an attempt to lessen the torque on their lumbar spine. The chance of injuring your back from doing this move is huge. And there are too many other ways to target your abs to take this risk.

WHAT TO DO INSTEAD: The double crunch. Lie on your back with your hands behind your head and your legs raised in the air and bent to 90 degrees. In one fluid movement lift your shoulder blades off the ground while bringing your knees toward your chest, return to the starting position, and repeat.

Double Crunch

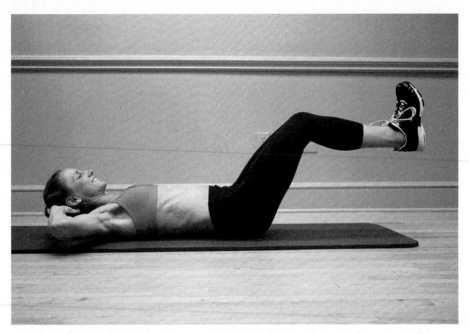

Lift your upper body off the floor while pulling your knees toward your chest.

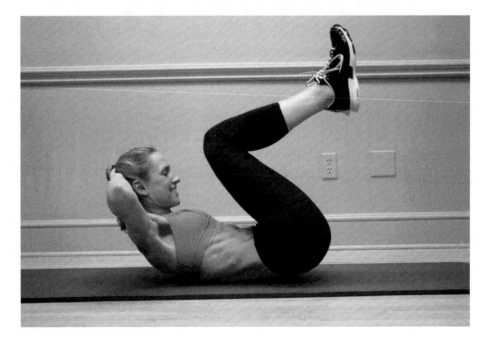

Upright Rows

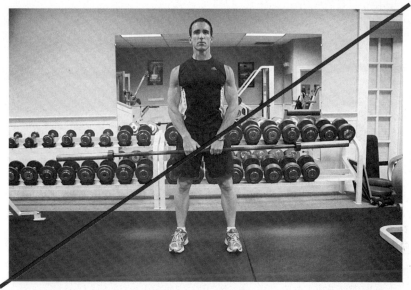

This exercise can strain the shoulder joint.

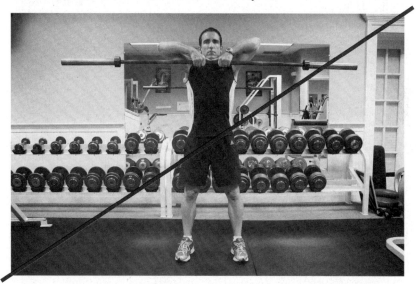

2. **UPRIGHT ROWS.** I'm not a fan of any kind of upright row, whether with barbells or a dumbbell. This shoulder exercise has you standing while holding weight against your legs with your arms straight and your hands close together. You pull the barbell straight up your body to the top of your chest, then lower it again.

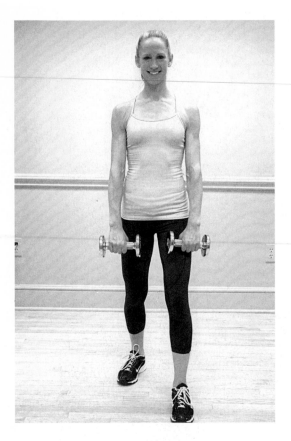
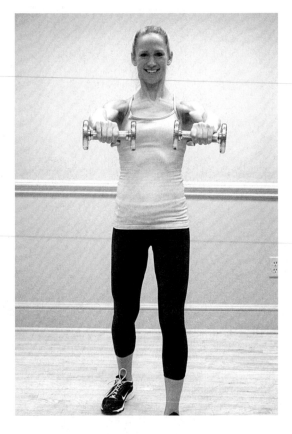

WHY IT'S BAD: This movement can stress the shoulder joint, leading to shoulder problems.

WHAT TO DO INSTEAD: Dumbbell front raises. This exercise targets the same shoulder muscles without compromising the integrity of the shoulder joint. In other words, it's a much safer exercise yet just as effective.

3. **LAT PULL-DOWNS BEHIND THE HEAD.** This exercise, so often pictured in fitness magazines, is another one that should be avoided.

> **WHY IT'S BAD:** Like the upright row, lat pull-downs behind the head can put the shoulder joint into an unfavorable position and lead to shoulder problems. Leave it out. You're not missing anything except the potential for a rotator cuff injury and time in a physical therapist's office. It feels awkward anyway.

Lat Pull-Downs—Bad

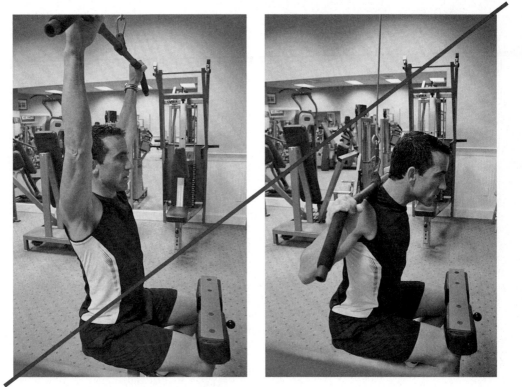

More bad strain on your shoulders.

WHAT TO DO INSTEAD: Lat pull-downs to the chest. This is a very simple modification without the negative impact on the shoulder joint. Keep the bar in front of your head rather than behind it, leaning back slightly and pulling it to the top of your chest.

Lat Pull-Downs—Good

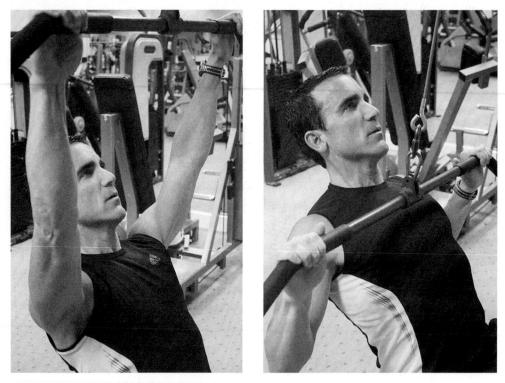

Focus on pulling from your back muscles.

Other Fun "Toys" Often Found in the Strength Training Area

1. **FOAM ROLLERS.** Long cylinders of foam, usually white, the primary use of which is to stretch out muscles, especially those of the lower body. You roll back and forth on them to loosen up tight muscles. Whether you are targeting your quadriceps, glutes, calves, or especially your "IT band," the foam roller is a fantastic way to loosen tight muscles.

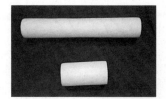

Ask a Trainer: What is the IT band?

It's a heck of a hard area to stretch. The IT, or iliotibial band is a layer of connective tissue on the outside of the leg extending from the hip to the knee. When the IT band is overly tight, it can lead to problems, including pain on the outside of the knee. If you've ever had tight IT bands, you know exactly where this band is.

2. **BALANCE BOARDS AND DISCS.** These are used to introduce instability to exercises such as squats, lunges, and push-ups, forcing the body to recruit different muscles, involve the core, and improve balance and coordination. They are especially helpful for rehabilitation purposes as well as improving sports performance.

Balance Boards

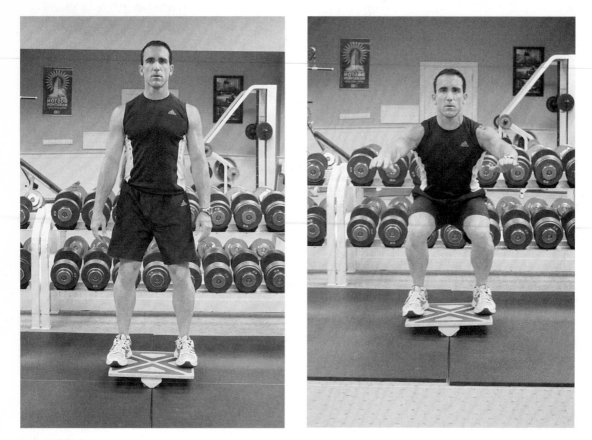

Squat down while trying to keep the board straight.

Balance Discs

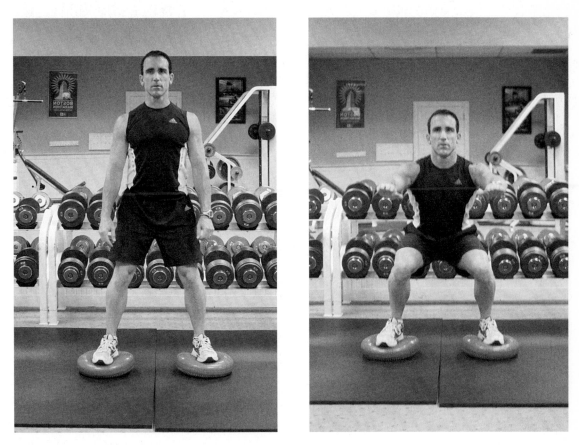

Unstable squats force your body to recruit more muscles.

3. **THE WHEEL.** Very old school and a former infomercial product, the wheel is simply a wheel with a handle on either side used to strengthen and tone the abs. You kneel down, place the wheel on the floor, and then push it away from you until your upper body is parallel to the floor; then you pull yourself back to the 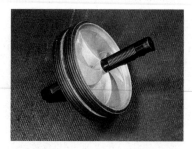 starting position. Anyone who has used the wheel knows it's not easy. You risk falling on your face if you're not strong enough. If you are seriously strong and daring, you can try to do the wheel while on your toes instead of your knees.

Ask a Trainer: What are plyometrics?

A higher-intensity type of exercise often utilized by athletes for sports conditioning, plyometrics involve rapid contractions of the muscles, blending power with speed. Often involving some kind of jumping movement, an example of a plyometric exercise would be jumping up and down off a box. As this type of exercise is high intensity, extra care must be taken when performing these movements. Plyometrics should be done only by people with a certain baseline of strength, after a thorough warm-up, and with special attention to proper form.

Bench Jump

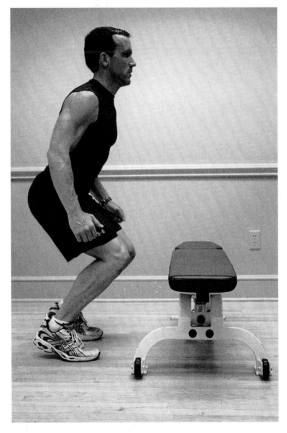 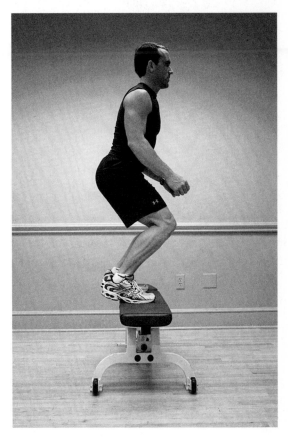

Jump your way to better fitness.

The Top Trainer Tricks for Building a Great Body

It may surprise you to learn that it doesn't matter whether you want a lean physique like a dancer or a massive, hulking frame like a bodybuilder; there are certain universal tricks that apply to all types of strength training, regardless of your goal. Apply these concepts, and you cannot fail!

1. **SLOW DOWN.** Too often you see people at the gym pumping through repetitions at breakneck speed. They throw weights around with little or no control. This is often due to their weights being too light or too heavy. Either way, the results are diminished, and the likelihood of injury is increased exponentially when exercises are done fast. Slow each repetition way down, the slower the better. Now, don't misunderstand me; you shouldn't go ridiculously slow (as one exercise fad proposed), just slow enough to be able to control the weight through the entire range of motion. If you need specific numbers, think of it as a slow count of two on the raising of the weight, then slightly slower on the down, or lowering, phase of the movement, a slow count of three. This leads to tip 2:

2. **BECOME KING TUT.** "TUT" stands for "time under tension." In strength training it means that we want to keep the tension on the muscle we are working for as long as possible. When we throw weights around, we have very little muscle TUT. When we slow down, the TUT increases dramatically. The better you get at developing your TUT skills, the greater your results will be. Know that this skill takes time to develop. It involves the recruitment of muscle fibers. The more experience you have lifting weights, the more muscle fibers you will be able to recruit. The more muscle fibers you recruit, the stronger and more toned you will be. You can develop this skill by focusing on the muscle you are working, slowing the movement down, and keeping the tension on that muscle from start to finish.

3. **ACCENTUATE THE NEGATIVE.** All these principles are interrelated. In order to slow down the exercises and focus on the muscle TUT, we also have to accentuate the "negative," or down, phase of the exercise. This is the part of the movement that so many people just "throw away." They allow gravity or momentum to take over, missing an essential component of the movement. Take the squat, for example. As most people squat down, they really just "fall," allowing gravity to move their body down toward the earth. They then work to raise their body, then "fall" all over again. This is incredibly ineffective, yet people do it with almost every exercise. Push-ups. Biceps curls. Leg press. This is the reason for the two-second/three-second rule I described earlier. By slowing the down part of each exercise, you will essentially double your results.

4. **MEN: LEGGO THE EGO.** And lift lighter weights—weights that don't require momentum and allow you to use good form. Unless you are a power lifter (I'm not sure too many power lifters will be reading this book, but if you are one, hey, thanks for buying it!), ego will keep you from reaching your goals. Ego will also get you hurt. Suck it up for an hour and go lighter. What are your true goals? To show off to the guys around you, or to look and feel your best? I can't tell you how many times I have been approached in the gym and asked if I were hurt. Sometimes people think that because I look strong yet am lifting lighter weights than they would expect, I must be hurt. On the contrary, it is by lifting lighter weights and constantly applying these principles that I have built the body I have. Time under tension, eliminating momentum, keeping good form: these can be done only with weights that you can control, that you move slowly and deliberately. By using lighter weights, you recruit more of the muscle fibers that you are trying to target. More muscle fibers equals more results. You increase the effectiveness of the exercise by "affecting" more of the muscle.

5. **REALIZE THAT YOUR MAIN GOAL IS TO FAIL.** To achieve as much failure as possible. Muscle failure, that is. You want to take your muscles to the

brink. Work them hard, but not too hard. The rule of thumb is that you want the final few repetitions to be difficult without losing your form. Remember the old "No pain, no gain" marketing campaign? Well, there was something to that. Pain is not the goal, but overloading your muscles is.

Trainer Tip: Maintain a "staggered stance."

When doing a standing exercise such as a biceps curl with a barbell or a front raise with dumbbells, use a staggered stance. This means putting one foot a few inches in front of the other. This foot position will help stabilize your body, minimizing the amount of swing or movement during the exercise. This added stability will help minimize your use of momentum, not only protecting your lower back from injury but also increasing the effectiveness of the exercise itself.

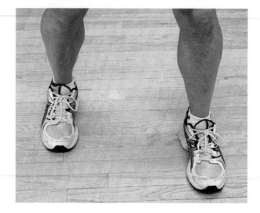

Lifting Lingo: The Overload Principle

One of the primary goals of strength training is to overload your muscles. This principle is quite simple: By overloading a muscle, you stress it. By stressing it, you break down the muscle tissue. By breaking down the muscle tissue, you force it to adapt. When it adapts, it rebuilds itself. When it rebuilds itself, the muscle becomes more toned and you become stronger.

If you do not provide enough of a stimulus to overload the muscle, adaptation will not take place. If adaptation does not take place, nothing changes. Make sense? That's why so many people fail to see results from their strength workouts; they do not work their muscles significantly enough to make their body change.

Ask a Trainer: Should I wear lifting gloves?

It's up to you. Lifting gloves are similar to the gloves used in golf or baseball. They most often come without fingers, and their primary use is to protect the hands against blisters and calluses. If you feel they help you with your workout, by all means wear them.

Rule 10: Don't Waste Time Standing Around Waiting to Use Equipment

I see this all the time: some guy who wants to use the leg press standing with his arms folded waiting for another guy to finish using it. That's a big no-no. You need to maximize your time at the gym. Instead of waiting idly for a machine, do the following.

1. Stretch.

2. Do jumping jacks.

3. Do an abdominal exercise.

4. Do a set of push-ups.

5. Go use another machine and come back.

The takeaway lesson is to do something and keep moving. Keep your heat rate elevated so you continue to burn calories. Use the opportunity to do something such as stretching that you wouldn't normally do. Even straying from your workout routine and doing one set of another exercise is beneficial; it will add much-needed variation to your workout.

Gym Etiquette: "Working in"

If there is a piece of equipment that someone is using and you also need to use, you can politely ask if you can "work in." What this means is that when she is done with her set, you then do a set, then she does, and so on. Wait to ask if you can work in until the person has completed a set, or, if you must ask while they are working out, wait until you have eye contact and the person doesn't look as if she is straining herself.

Ask a Trainer: Do I have to let someone work in? What if I don't want to?

There is no rule that says you have to let a person work in. There is also no rule that you have to hold the elevator for someone or give up a seat on a bus for an elderly person. But they are nice things to do, and you don't end up looking like a jerk.

Having spent decades in the gym experiencing and observing bad behavior on the gym floor, I am so excited to finally be able to vent. I'm sure many of you regular gymgoers will be able to relate to these and will probably have a few additions of your own.

More Bad Etiquette While Strength Training

1. **YELLING.** I have a very simple rule of thumb. If you have to yell, it's too heavy. It's also really annoying for all of the people around you. Listen, I'm all for overloading the muscles and working hard. Occasional grunts and groans are acceptable. But nonstop hollering is not okay. Either take off a few plates or take it down a few decibels.

2. **HOGGING A MACHINE.** I just discussed the concept of working in. Though it's good etiquette to agree to do so, it's not mandatory. What is unacceptable is sitting on a machine such as a shoulder press machine while chatting away, reading a magazine, or, worse yet, using your BlackBerry or iPhone. I can't tell you how many guys I now see at the gym using one of these while they are working out. It's ridiculous. Leave the phone in your locker. That leads to the next bad etiquette rule.

3. **TALKING ON A CELL PHONE.** Really? Do I even have to include this one? Unfortunately, I do. There are a bunch of chuckleheads out there who think we want to listen to them chatting up their friends while we are trying to get a workout in. Guess what? We don't. The lack of consciousness of some people is amazing: I can't tell you how many times I have witnessed someone talking on a cell phone within inches of a sign that prohibits their use in the gym.

4. **"SAVING" A PIECE OF EQUIPMENT.** I used to go to a certain gym to work out on Saturday mornings. It was packed. One guy would do a set of biceps curls on a bench, then leave his towel on it and the dumbbells alongside while he went across the gym to do crunches, lat pull-downs, whatever, then return five minutes later to do another set of biceps curls. Not okay.

5. **STANDING RIGHT IN FRONT OF THE DUMBBELL RACK WHILE DOING AN EXERCISE.** You know the guy. The one who pulls the fifty-pound dumbbells off of the rack, then stands an inch away, doing shoulder shrugs while staring at himself in the mirror. Meanwhile, you'd love to use the forty-pound dumbbells, but he's blocking them. Proper etiquette dictates that you pick up the dumbbells and back away from the rack. There should be at least enough space for a person to walk comfortably in between you and the rack.

6. **NOT PUTTING YOUR WEIGHTS BACK.** Whether it's dumbbells or plates on a machine, when you are finished with it, put it back. There is nothing more annoying than having to take a stack of forty-five-pound plates off of the leg press that someone has left behind. This is one of the biggest pet peeves around. If you use it, put it away.

Rule 11: Start Each Workout by Doing One Exercise You Hate

The exercises you hate are the ones that will have a big impact on your body. You don't like them, you never do them; therefore they will provide a huge positive "shock" to your body. Do just one exercise you dislike to start each workout. If you wait until the end of your workout, you won't do it. Do just one. Small steps bring about big changes.

STRENGTH TRAINING MYTHS

1. **YOU CAN TURN FAT INTO MUSCLE AND VICE VERSA.** Nope. A fat cell is a fat cell, and a muscle cell is a muscle cell, never the twain shall meet. Muscles grow bigger through exercise and decrease in size when you stop working out for an extended period of time. Fat cells also grow bigger and smaller due to changes in diet, but one never turns into the other. The old former bodybuilders who look horrible and fat? That's not muscle that has turned into fat. It's just fat.

2. **YOU SHOULD WEAR A WEIGHT BELT.** Not unless you are a power lifter or someone lifting big, and I mean big, poundage. Studies on weight belts indicate that those who use them do so at the expense of building core strength. The belt becomes a "crutch." When you use one, you don't learn how to stabilize your body on its own. This can lead to injury when lifting without a belt, especially during everyday activities. It's better to learn how to stabilize the abdominal muscles when lifting while building core strength as well.

3. **SQUATS ARE BAD FOR YOUR KNEES.** Nope. *Bad* squats are bad for your knees. Good squats are one of the best exercises not only for strengthening the muscles around your knees but for toning the lower body as well. But you need to do them right. Here are some tips on how to do a perfect squat.

   - The first movement should be from your hips: move your hips back as if you were going to sit down in a chair.
   - Keep your chest up and pointed forward. Many people drop their head and chest down toward the floor after they swing their hips

back. Look straight ahead as you begin to squat down, keeping your chest pointed ahead and not at the floor.

- Keep your weight on your heels. If your weight is on your toes, you will put undue stress on your knees.

- Keep your knees behind your toes. Better yet, try to keep them over your ankles. Again, doing this involves keeping your weight on your heels. The more your knees move forward doing a squat, the more pressure there is on your patella or kneecap. You want to minimize the stress on your knees.

4. **SQUATS WILL MAKE WOMEN'S LEGS BIG.** Nope. So many women avoid doing one of the most effective lower-body exercises because of this ridiculous myth. I have listened to countless women tell me how they "just had to stop doing squats" because they legs "got huge." Usually after just a few sessions. If it were only that easy! Women simply don't have the testosterone necessary to get big legs. They may "feel" that their legs are bigger. They may be tighter, or more sore from squats, but they definitely are not "huge" as a result. Not even close. Remember, exercise will not make a woman huge, overeating will. And not doing your workouts.

5. **DO THE WORKOUTS IN THE MAGAZINES, AND YOU WILL LOOK JUST LIKE THE GUYS INSIDE.** This one really drives me nuts. So many men's magazines leave out the single most important ingredient needed to look like the guy flexing with the perfect body: drugs. No matter how faithfully you follow the workout routines, unless you use steroids, human growth hormone, diuretics, whatever, you will never look like the Adonis in the article. The magazines are setting you up for failure. Does this mean you can't sculpt an amazing body without drugs? Absolutely not. You most certainly can. You just won't ever look as big or as ripped as the majority of those guys without significant pharmaceutical help.

Rule 12: The Best Lower-Body Exercise Is the Squat!

The squat is one of the most effective exercises for toning the lower body. It's simple, you can do it anywhere, and you can modify it in an infinite number of ways to keep the results coming. On a BOSU ball, with a barbell, while holding a medicine ball: there are innumerable ways to change a squat. This exercise is one of the top tools in every great trainer's exercise arsenal.

MORE LIFTING LINGO

1. **REPETITIONS.** This refers to how many times you do a movement within a set. So "two sets of 10 biceps curls" means 10 repetitions.

2. **SETS.** Back to the biceps example, "two sets of 10 biceps curls" means you will lift the weight 10 times, rest, then do it a second time. That's two "sets." You would be amazed at how many people get the terms "sets" and "reps" confused.

3. **SUPERSET.** This is two exercises performed back to back with minimal rest in between. Though supersets can involve any two muscle groups, they are often done with opposing muscle groups: biceps, then triceps; chest, then back.

4. **SPLIT ROUTINE.** This means you split up your workout. Instead of doing a full-body workout each time, you might do chest back and triceps on one day, back and biceps the second day, and legs the third. Split routines are generally used by people who want to strength train five to six days per week, lifting heavier weights, and are looking to significantly increase their muscle size. Bodybuilders do split routines.

5. **FAILURE.** This refers to failure of a muscle to be able to do another repetition with good form. When you have reached this point, you have completely fatigued the muscle.

6. **DROP SET.** This means starting with a heavy weight and decreasing the weight for each successive set; for instance, doing 100 pounds on the machine chest press for 12 repetitions, then 90 pounds for 12, 80 pounds for 12, and so on. You can also go to fatigue instead of doing a specified number of repetitions. One arm workout I like to do with

clients is "running the rack" of dumbbells for biceps curls. This may include doing 40-pound dumbbell curls until you cannot do any more (keeping good form), then doing 35 pounds until exhaustion, 30 pounds, 25, and so on. By the time you get to 5 pounds, you can barely do 3 reps.

7.   **PYRAMID SET.** This means progressing from lighter weights with a greater number of repetitions in the first set to heavier weights with fewer repetitions in subsequent sets. So for the bench press you might do 12 reps of 150 pounds, then 8 reps of 175 pounds, 6 reps of 200 pounds, 4 reps of 225, and finish with 2 reps of 250 pounds.

8.   **REVERSE PYRAMID SET.** This is the same as a pyramid set, only you begin with heavier weight and fewer repetitions and progress to lighter weights with more repetitions.

9.   **SPOT.** This means to assist a person while he does an exercise, standing ready to help raise the weight so that the person can do additional repetitions if he so desires and/or lift the weight when he is unable to do another. The most common time to spot a person is during the bench press, but you can also spot shoulder presses, squats, and other exercises.

10. **FORCED REPETITION.** This means helping a person do another repetition when he is unable to do it on his own. Forced repetitions are done by people who are looking to significantly increase their size and/or strength.

Gym Etiquette: Spotting

Think of it as supervising someone as he does an exercise. You are there to help him if and when he needs help. Take a barbell bench press, for example. This is a common exercise that calls for a spot. You stand behind the person's head, ready to provide assistance when necessary. It sounds pretty basic, but there are certain subtleties involved. You need to know the intricacies if you plan to spend time in the gym, as follows.

1. If asked by someone to spot him, common courtesy dictates that you say yes. It takes only a few seconds, and if you need a spot, someone would help you out.

2. Take a look at how much weight the person is trying to lift. If it's too much for you to assist with, say so! If you're not able to help bring the weight back up, he could get really hurt. Be honest with him. Say you'd like to help but you don't think you're strong enough.

3. Begin by asking how many reps the person is trying for. This will give you an idea of when you may need to help out.

4. Some people get extremely annoyed if you help them before they think they need the help (the operative word here being "think"). They want "full credit" for the exercise and don't want any assistance unless absolutely necessary. You should also clarify this with the person beforehand. After you ask how many reps he is trying to do, ask if he wants help with the last few. If he says no, you shouldn't help him until you're absolutely, positively sure that he can't complete the rep. Let him struggle. Let him sweat. When he screams for help, then help.

5. Take spotting seriously. Pay complete attention to what you are doing. Stand at the ready to help at a second's notice. You can keep your hands a few inches from the bar, out of the way but ready to grab it in a split second. For something like the bench press, I like to put my index fingers under the bar when the person starts to struggle. This way he can see that I'm not really assisting him but am ready to grab the bar if he needs me to.

6. Offer a few words of encouragement. When you see the person start to struggle, throw out a few encouragers to help motivate him. A simple "Come on!" "Push!" or "You can do it!" is helpful and often appreciated.

Trainer Tip: Hand placement in a push-up is key.

I am often asked if it is better to have your hands positioned wide or close together during a push-up. Both are correct. The difference is that the closer your hands are, the more it becomes predominantly an arm exercise, specifically targeting the triceps. The wider you space your hands during a push-up, the more the chest muscles are involved.

Ask a Trainer: How much does the bar weigh?

The long silver-colored bar most commonly used for the bench press weighs 45 pounds.

Trainer Tip: Do push-ups hurt your wrists? Do them on dumbbells.

The position a push-up puts the wrists in can be painful to many people. Placing two dumbbells on the floor and holding on to them while you perform the movement will often take the pain away completely.

Abdominals: The Elusive Six-Pack

Yes, we're going to talk about them again. Flat abs. Everybody wants them. Few have them after age thirty. And the age at which people lose their flat stomach is getting younger and younger. The desire to have a six-pack is so strong that it's a billion-dollar industry. There is a seemingly infinite amount of late-night infomercials, DVDs, diet drugs, and the like that promise to deliver perfectly flat abs if you just use the products.

It's not gonna happen.

As I said earlier, getting flat abs is something like 80 percent diet. Now, this is not a scientific number, just an anecdote based on years and years of training clients and working out. Most qualified fitness professionals will quote you roughly the same percentage.

This does not mean that you are off the hook for doing abdominal exercises. You still have to do them. I just want you to be aware of what it truly takes to get flat abs. Yes, you have to work to achieve them. But it can be done. Just know that it's diet first, cardio second, and abdominal exercises third; something like 80 percent diet, 10 percent cardio, and 10 percent ab exercises.

Once again, I break the abdominals into three different regions: the rectus abdominis, or "six-pack"; the obliques or side abs; and the lower abdominals. You should focus on targeting all three of these areas. If you really want to sculpt your midsection, you need to exercise all three of these areas effectively.

There are certain simple rules on how to effectively target these three parts of your abs:

1. **FLEX YOUR SPINE.** Working the middle of your stomach is very straightforward. You want to flex your spine forward, by doing a regular crunch, for example. This is the primary movement to target your six-pack.

Abs Flex

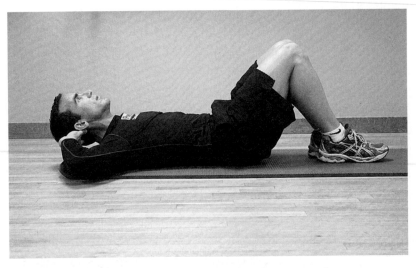

Lifting your upper body off the floor flexes your spine.

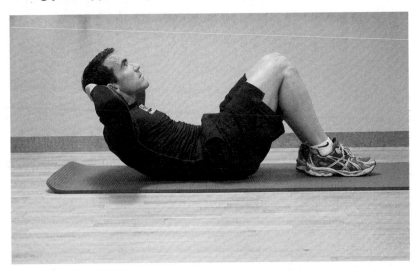

2. **TWIST.** To sculpt the obliques, the sides of your abs, you want to rotate your upper body and perform twisting movements.

Abs Twist

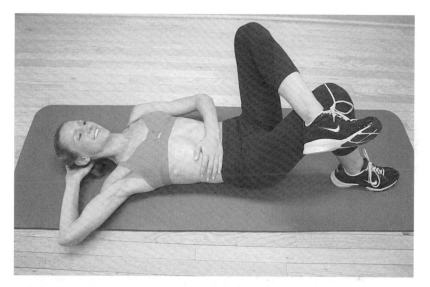

Bring your elbow toward your opposite knee.

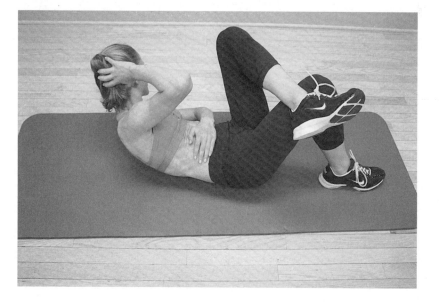

3. **USE YOUR LEGS.** Once you start to involve your legs in an abdominal movement, you engage the muscle fibers of the lower abdominals. If targeting the six-pack involves spinal flexion, bringing your upper body toward your legs, focusing on the lower abs involves bringing your legs toward your upper body. A reverse crunch, bicycle crunches, and hanging leg lifts are three examples of involving the legs to work the lower part of your abdomen.

Abs Leg Pull

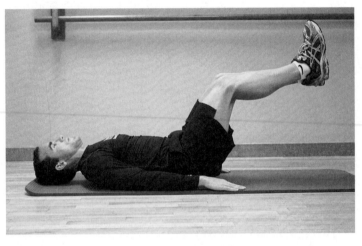

Raising your legs helps to activate your lower abs.

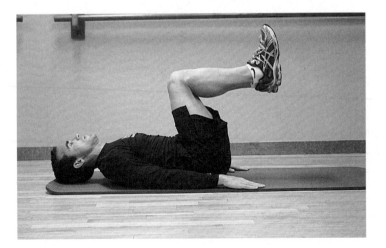

Trainer Tip: Do a reverse pelvic tilt.

Your body has something known as a lordotic curve. When you are standing upright, it is the natural curvature found in your lower back. When you lie on your back to do abdominal exercises, especially lower abdominal moves whereby you lift your legs off the ground, you want to get rid of this curve to protect your lower back. You do this by performing what is known as a "reverse pelvic tilt," in essence pressing your lower back into the floor, eliminating the space between your lower back and the ground. Lifting your legs while on your back can put a large amount of torque on the lower back region. This can lead to injury; performing a reverse pelvic tilt can help minimize the risk.

Trainer Tip: When correctly performing a reverse pelvic tilt, you should not be able to slide your hand between your lower back and the floor.

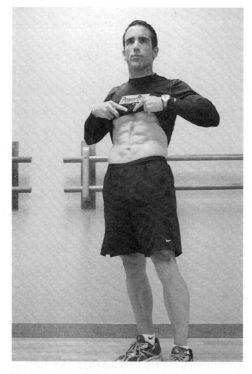

These are not painted on.

Ask a Trainer: Can I work out my abs every day?

Ask ten trainers this question, and five will probably say yes, five will say no. The ones who say no will base it on the rule about not working the same muscle two days in a row. Those who say you can do abs on consecutive days will talk about how they are postural muscles and their characteristics allow them to be worked out more often.

I fall in between the two thought processes. Though I don't believe you should work out your abs seven days a week, I do believe you can do ab exercises on consecutive days. I think that doing some kind of core exercise five days a week is a recipe for amazing abs. You still want two days off per week to allow the abdominal muscles to rebuild themselves, but you can crunch away two or more days in a row. So you can do abs on Monday and Tuesday, take Wednesday off, do them again Thursday, Friday, and Saturday, and take Sunday off.

Years ago, when I was just starting out in New York City, an up-and-coming actor hired me as his trainer. His primary goal was to get a six-pack. He had read that Antonio Sabato Jr. was doing one thousand crunches a day. He decided that if Antonio was doing one thousand, he should do two thousand. And he wanted me to do them with him. So the actor paid me to do two thousand crunches per session with him. I would never do this with a client today, but I was very green and he paid really well!

We did sets of fifty, about forty different abdominal exercises. This, as you can guess, was a huge waste of time. Doing a few hundred per session was all we really needed, and even that was probably too much for him. He would have been much better off doing a maximum of ten to fifteen minutes of core exercises and spending the rest of the time burning calories through cardio.

Here is a more advanced way to structure your weekly ab workouts. It breaks each session down by abdominal region:

MONDAY	TUESDAY	WEDNESDAY	THURSDAY	FRIDAY	SATURDAY	SUNDAY
Rectus abdominis	Obliques	Lower abs	Rectus abdominis	Obliques	Lower abs	REST

Ask a Trainer: What is the absolute best exercise to flatten your stomach?

The bicycle crunch.

Rule 13: The Bicycle Crunch Is One of the Most Effective Abdominal Exercises

In laboratory tests the bicycle crunch was found to produce a large amount of muscle activation, making it an extremely effective tummy-toning move, one that requires no equipment. Every good abdominal routine should include the bicycle crunch.

Bicycle Crunch

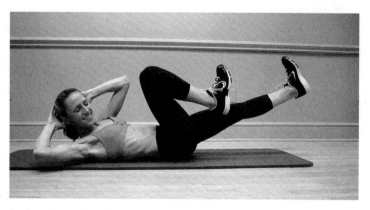

Alternate bringing your elbow toward your opposite knee.

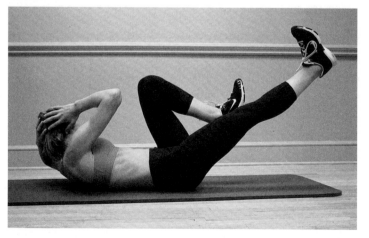

Trainer Tip: Doing crunches with your hands behind your head is slightly harder than doing them with your hands folded across your chest.

This has to do with the concepts of moment arms, distance from the axis of rotation, torque, and more—cool things for an exercise physiologist to study but probably really boring for you. All you need to know is that putting your hands behind your head will make a regular crunch more difficult than keeping them in front of you.

Crunch Hands Behind

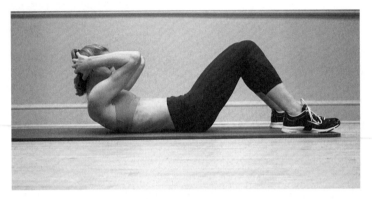

A little harder.

Crunch Hands Across

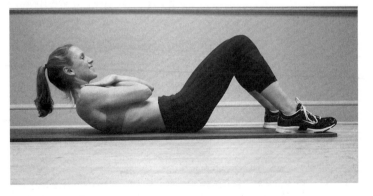

A little easier.

Rule 14: Abdominal "Dos" and "Don'ts"

1. **DO:** Go slowly during your ab exercises. Focus on eliminating momentum.

   DON'T: Hook your feet under anything like a bar or piece of furniture. By securing your feet, you start to involve your hip flexor muscles instead of focusing on your abdominals.

2. **DO:** Remember to breathe. I know, I know, it sounds really dumb to have to remind people to breathe, but you'd be amazed at how many people hold their breath when doing core exercises.

   DON'T: Make the ab exercise too complicated. Keep it simple. By adding too many components, such as stability balls, medicine balls, and hanging positions, it becomes increasingly difficult to initiate the movement from the muscles you are trying to target.

3. **DO:** Mix up your routine. Just like every other muscle in your body, your abdominals need variation in order to change. There are so many people who have been doing the same abdominal exercises for years. Their routine has not changed, and neither have their abs as a result.

   DON'T: Hold weights that are too heavy during a crunch. I see people with twenty-five-pound plates across their chests struggling to do a regular crunch. Yes, you want to make your exercises challenging, but not overly challenging to the point that form is comprised and the potential for injury becomes great. Rather than using weight, try slowing the move down and pausing at the top. You will be shocked at how much harder that makes the exercise. And how much more effective.

More Quick Crunch Tips

1. Keep your chin off of your chest when doing a crunch. Imagine that there is an invisible tennis ball between your chin and your chest.

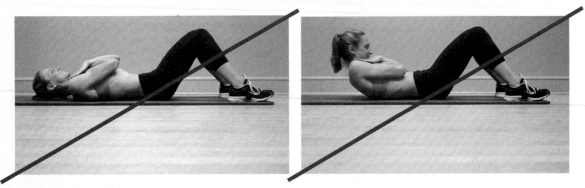

Bad head position.

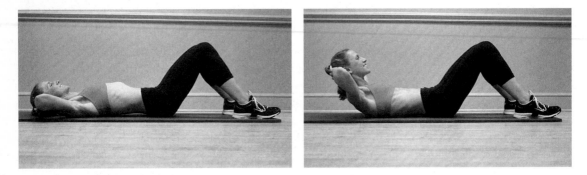

Good head position.

2. Look at a spot on the ceiling above you. This will help keep your head in the right position.

3. Keep your abs flat throughout the movement. This is difficult for many people to do. You are not "sucking in" your gut muscles; you are "engaging" them. I like to describe it like this: Imagine a child is about to punch you in the stomach. The same way you would tighten your abs in reaction to that is the way you should keep those muscles throughout ab exercises.

If you are new to free weights or machines, take pride in getting through your first workout. It's not easy. You think everyone is looking at you. You often feel awkward, clumsy, and pretty darn weak. Realize that *everyone* felt that way as well when he or she started. You are not alone.

It will get better. Much better. And fast. I promise. First, I want you to take pride in the fact that you got through the workout. Way to go! You are on your way to BEATING THE GYM and seeing results you only dreamed were possible.

Second, I want you to realize that you will probably be sore, *really* sore afterward. And not the day afterward, but quite often two days afterward. This is known as DOMS, an abbreviation for "delayed-onset muscle soreness." It happens to everyone who starts a fitness program or returns to one after an extended time off. It has to do with the breakdown of the muscle fibers. What I want you to understand is that you will *not* be that sore each time you work out. In fact, each time you work out, you will be a little less sore afterward. You will never again be as sore as you were after the first session, and soon you will feel great after your workouts.

So don't let the soreness stop you. Think of it as your body reshaping itself. Because it is.

Fit Myth: Soreness after a strength workout is caused by lactic acid.

Nope. It is due to microscopic tears in the muscle tissue. When you exercise, you break the tissue down, and when the muscle rebuilds itself, you become stronger and more toned. Research has shown that it is specifically the eccentric, or lowering, part of the exercise that is the primary cause of this soreness. So lowering the weight during a biceps curl is making you more sore than the lifting and squeezing of the muscle.

Trainer Tip: What should you do about DOMS?

Often the soreness is accompanied by tight muscles. Doing a low-level aerobic activity such as walking can actually help loosen you up and feel better. Soaking in a hot bath can also minimize the aftereffects. Taking an anti-inflammatory can help lessen the pain. Realize, however, that the true cure for the soreness associated with DOMS is time. It will go away in a day or two.

4

Not All Classes Are Going to Make You Sweat: The Skinny on What Classes to Take and Which to Avoid

Zumba. Yoga. Spinning. Mat Pilates. Boot camp. Kickboxing. Stripper pole. Group exercise classes are a huge part of the gym experience. But figuring out which class is right for you and which class will actually help you BEAT THE GYM can be a challenge. I've taught hundreds of classes over the years, from spinning to total body conditioning, boot camp to biathlon, core conditioning and more. I highly recommend them as a supplement and a fun alternative to both the cardio and strength training machines. As I have said over and over, you have to feel the exercise to know you are getting something out of it, but the good classes can get you fit while being exciting and enjoyable enough to get your mind off the burn.

I realize that classes can be really intimidating. It seems as though everyone in them is superfit. You think that you can never learn the routines. And if you are possibly able to learn the steps or moves, you will surely die trying to keep up. Well, once again, all the others in the class were beginners at one time. I don't care how fit they are, they too were nervous walking in the door. You can do it. You just have to walk in and be willing to try.

I was freaked out before my first Spinning class. I too was a "newbie." I didn't know what I was doing. After just a class or two I soon realized that there was no reason to be nervous. And that it was really fun.

Trainer Tip: People are *not* staring at you. They are too busy staring at *themselves*.

This is a really important point when it comes to beating the gym, possibly *the* most important rule, especially when it comes to taking classes. People are so self-conscious when it comes to exercising in public. They mistakenly believe that everyone is going to be watching them, that all eyes will be focused on them, so they avoid trying new things. This is a huge mistake. Take it from someone who has spent his life in the gym: people are way too busy worrying about themselves to be paying any attention to you.

So get over it. And get into that class you have always wanted to take.

Trainer Tip: Classes are *not* for women only

For many years men were hesitant to take classes. It wasn't considered masculine. We were too cool: too cool to work out with strangers, too cool to have someone tell us what to do. It was the rare class that had any male participants, and if there were men in there, there were but a few.

Well, all that has changed. Men take spin, yoga, Pilates, boot camp, and cardio kickboxing. You name it, men now take it. We have realized that these classes are no longer for women only. Men have put aside their egos and realized that classes are really fun and really effective. Again, as humans we tend to do what we are good at. This approach does not help us work on our weaknesses and can help magnify our imbalances and weak links. When we take classes that challenge us, engage in workouts that are a little bit outside our "comfort zone," that is when we really start to see our bodies change and improve for the better.

Many people join a gym just to take classes. There are several reasons classes can play such a huge part of achieving your fitness goals:

1. **MOTIVATION.** Most people don't like working out alone. Suffering with a whole bunch of people who are experiencing the same pain makes it much more tolerable. There is power in numbers.

2. **INSTRUCTION.** Good instructors are trained to deliver a safe, effective workout. They have studied their craft. They know what they are doing. They will push you to your limits without hurting you. Yoga instructors are required to have hundreds of hours of training. Many group cycling teachers are also accomplished cyclists or triathletes. Take advantage of their experience and education by taking their classes.

3. **GOAL-SETTING COMPONENT.** Effective goal setting is essential to hitting your fitness goals. Exercise classes can be a big part of this. Classes provide you with a concrete day and time for your workout. This may seem unimportant, but it is a powerful component of a long-term fitness plan. One common goal-setting strategy I use with clients is something like "I will go to two Spinning and one total body conditioning class every week." These are definitive goals that work. You know what you have to do. You know when you have to do it. And, at the end of the week, you know whether or not you've hit your goal.

4. **VARIATION.** Look at any gym's group exercise offerings, and you will be amazed at the wide selection of classes. Stretching, strength training, cardiovascular exercise, and many variations of all of these. As I have repeated over and over throughout the book, variation is one of the keys to your success. Challenge yourself and your body by taking a wide variety of classes. The more types of classes you take, the greater will be your results.

Rule 1: A Class Will Not "Take the Place of" the Wrong Thing

This is the elephant in the room. But I have to be honest if I want you to succeed and achieve all your fitness goals. Here goes:

- Yoga cannot take the place of your strength training workout.

- Power yoga will not take the place of your cardio workout.

- Pilates cannot take the place of your strength training workout.

- Bikram yoga will not take the place of your cardio workout.

- Boot camp class will not take the place of your cardio workout.

Though all these classes are a great part of an overall fitness program, too many people use them to try to cut corners. They are only cheating themselves. Here's how I would break down the classes by their true primary training effect:

CARDIO	STRENGTH TRAINING	STRENGTH/CARDIO COMBO*	MIND/BODY/OTHER
Spinning	Kettlebells	Boot camp	Yoga
Jump rope	TRX suspension training	Kickboxing	Pilates
Biathlon	Total body conditioning	Boxing	Tai chi
Zumba		Tabata	Yogilates
		Rebounding	IntenSati
		Insanity	

*These strength/cardio classes deliver a little of both but are not enough cardio or enough strength training to take the place of either one.

Some classes, such as kickboxing, have both a strength and a cardiovascular component. The newer to exercise you are, the greater the effects will be. You are doing yourself a huge disservice, however, by taking a few boot camp classes per week and thinking that you don't need to do any other cardio.

Disclaimer: Because there is so much variation in how instructors design their workouts, different classes with the same name can deliver markedly different training effects. One boot camp class might be primarily strength training moves with a lot of standing around in between. Another class, also called boot camp, may involve nonstop movement and cardio stations, with your heart rate significantly elevated throughout the entire workout.

Note that the "Strength/Cardio Combo" column has the most classes in it. This is because many group exercise classes do elevate your heart rate and provide certain strength training components. It is possible to take a wide variety of classes and get into great shape doing so. Just realize once again that your heart is a muscle, one that needs a significant amount of steady-state exercise at an elevated intensity.

Once again, I will return to one of the main themes of this book and the "secrets" of being fit for life: variation. Mix it up. Take some classes.

Rule 2: Classes Are Not for Women Only. Get Over It, Guys

COMMON MISTAKES TO AVOID WHEN TAKING CLASSES

1. **DOING ONE CLASS ONLY.** As human beings we tend to do what we like to
    do. And what we are good at. This works for only so long. I am forever
    running into people who are simply rabid about the new exercise class
    they are taking. "Tom, I *love* Spinning! I do it six days a week! Sometimes
    two classes in one day!" They are so enthusiastic about their new exercise
    routine that they have forsaken everything else. Three things inevitably
    happen as a result:

    ■   They plateau and stop seeing results.

    ■   They become injured. Running, Spinning, the elliptical machine, you name
        it—any repetitive motion done exclusively, no matter how healthful, will lead
        to musculoskeletal problems over time.

    ■   They get burned out. We all know such people or have been one of them
        ourselves. You throw yourself completely into a hot new exercise routine,
        only to loathe the very thought of it several months later. The sad part is,
        many people then cut those classes out forever.

2. **STUDYING WITH ONLY ONE INSTRUCTOR.** Not only do we tend to do what
    we like to do and are good at, we also do it only with whom we like. A
    great instructor is worth his or her weight in gold. When you find one, be
    thankful. Just be sure to try out other instructors as well. The variation will
    challenge your body in different ways and keep the routine from getting
    stale.

3. **AVOIDING A CLASS BECAUSE YOU THINK YOU'RE NOT READY.** I have
    listened to so many people who believe they are not fit enough to take
    a certain class. They stare in through the windows at the members
    Spinning, or taking yoga, or kickboxing, never trying it out because they
    think they can't do it. I don't care what your level of fitness is or what
    the class is, you can do it. Everyone in that class was a beginner at one
    time. Please do not let your fear of the unknown keep you from trying

out a great new exercise routine. If you are worried about trying out a new routine, speak with the instructor before or after the class. Tell the instructor that you are new and want to take the class. A good instructor will tell you how to get started: what specific class to take, where to position yourself in the studio, how to modify the routine if necessary, and so on.

GROUP CLASS ETIQUETTE

1. **KNOW YOUR PLACE.** When taking a class for the first time, realize that regular classgoers ("groupies," if you will) can be extremely territorial. Take "their" particular spin bike or their particular spot in the studio, and they might very well fight you to the death. I watched as one woman literally dragged another off her bike in my spin class. To avoid a potential fracas, wait a minute or two after class starts and let the regulars position themselves. You can also ask the teacher where you should situate yourself.

2. **KEEP THE SINGING AND SHOUTS TO A MINIMUM.** You may or may not have heard the story, but there was a lawsuit recently wherein one spin class member threw another off of his bike, allegedly injuring him. He was not tossed because he had taken his bike, as I observed in my class, but because he was "woo-ing" (see "Workout Word").

3. **GET TO CLASS ON TIME.** Most gyms have a rule about entering class late; usually the limit is five minutes or so after class has started. It's distracting to the class, to the instructor, and if the class is a popular one and you reserved a spot, the spot will often be given to someone else. Get to class a few minutes early.

4. **DON'T LEAVE EARLY.** Unless you have a very good reason for doing so, do not leave class before it is over. Like coming in late, it's distracting to both the class and the instructor. If you know ahead of time that you have to leave a few minutes early, common courtesy dictates that you let the instructor know beforehand. He or she may ask you to take a spot near the exit so you can slip out quietly. Honor the instructor's wishes.

5. **WIPE DOWN YOUR AREA AFTERWARD.** Whether it's a spin bike or your nine square feet in the aerobics room, wipe your sweat from the area at the end of class. Some gyms have maintenance people for this, but not all of them clean up after every class. Even if they do, show some manners and clean up after yourself as well. Those guys don't get paid enough as it is.

Rule 3: I Don't Care How Good a Singer You Are. No One Wants to Hear You Do It in Class

I have taught many a spin class over the years where one or more people have decided to sing along during the workout. "Paradise by the Dashboard Light" would be blaring for our final round of intervals when suddenly someone would think she was back in a bar in college, holding a beer bottle like a microphone while signing drunkenly to her friends. I am all for getting into the workout and having a great time, but express yourself through the workout, your intensity, not your voice.

Workout Word: Woo-er

A "woo-er" is someone who spontaneously yells out during an exercise class with a sound that resembles something like "Woo!" Teachers have been known to "woo," and class members will often "woo" in response. Think of it as something along the lines of Spinners speaking in tongues.

1. **DON'T WEAR INAPPROPRIATE ATTIRE.** This rule is violated daily in gyms all across the country and around the world. First, spandex is a privilege, not a right. Especially for men. If you have to stuff yourself into it or it leaves little to the imagination, it's not okay to wear it in public. Also, if your favorite shorts or shirt has a dank sweat smell permanently "baked" into it, it's time to let it go. Throw it away. No one wants to be inhaling that odor mere inches from you in a small, unventilated room. Finally, dress appropriately for the decade. Guys, it's not okay to wear those Thomas Magnum–length shorts from the eighties anymore. And ladies, the Jane Fonda unitard should come out only on Halloween.

Quick Class Descriptions

Here are a few common classes and brief descriptions of what they generally involve.

1. **SPINNING.** This training method was created by the cyclist Jonathan "Johnny G" Goldberg as a way to train indoors. He opened his first Spinning center in California in the 1980s, and since then this group cycling class has exploded in popularity. Class participants work out on specially designed stationary bikes as an instructor leads them through a choreographed routine set to music.

2. **YOGA.** This is a tough one to give a short definition for. The term "Yoga" comes from the Sanskrit word *yuj*, meaning "to yoke, unite, or join." Yoga is a mind-body exercise routine that is much more than just a simple series of movements. In its simplest definition, yoga is a series of postures that is used as a form of exercise. People often use yoga to increase flexibility, for meditation purposes, and to build a specific type of strength.

3. **PILATES.** Originally developed during the First World War by Joseph Pilates to help prisoners of war stay fit, this exercise routine soon became a favorite conditioning method for dancers and is now experiencing widespread popularity. There are specific machines, including the Cadillac and Reformer, on which a teacher guides a client through a series of exercises. There is also mat Pilates, an exercise routine often done in groups, that involves little or no equipment. Pilates is said to increase core strength, flexibility, and body awareness.

4. **ZUMBA.** Created in the 1990s by the dancer and choreographer Alberto "Beto" Perez, Zumba is a dance-type workout involving Latin and international music.

5. **CORE CONDITIONING.** These classes specifically target the abdominals and lower back. Usually just thirty minutes in length, core conditioning classes are great for those trying to flatten their stomachs, improve

their sports performance, rehabilitate lower back issues, or prevent lower back pain in the future.

6. **BOOT CAMP.** Born out of the workouts performed by the military, boot camp classes involve a drill instructor, or DI, taking a class through a series of exercises. Though there is a wide variety of these classes, boot camp often involves people being taken through a series of exercise "stations" with little or no rest in between. Boot camp classes can involve various pieces of basic equipment (rope ladders, cones, steps, and so on) and are generally known for being challenging workouts.

7. **TABATA.** This class is named for the Japanese researcher Dr. Izumi Tabata, who studied the effects of high-intensity interval training, found it to have incredible cardiovascular results, and developed an exercise protocol involving just that. A Tabata interval cycle is just four minutes in length. It involves twenty seconds of all-out effort followed by ten seconds of rest, repeated eight times for a total of four minutes. Tabata group exercise classes have sprung up that incorporate this twenty-second/ten-second interval format to deliver an extremely intense workout.

8. **TOTAL-BODY CONDITIONING.** This is yet another class that differs greatly from club to club and instructor to instructor, but generally speaking a total-body conditioning class is a full-body workout routine involving weights. I used to teach one where each person had several sets of dumbbells, a step, and a mat. We would do all of the basic upper and lower-body exercises, abdominals, and even short cardio bursts. These classes can also use body bars, medicine balls, and other basic pieces of equipment.

9. **YOGILATES.** A blend of yoga and Pilates. Think core exercises, stretching, and isometric strength moves.

10. **KETTLEBELLS.** Supposedly invented in Russia and extremely popular in Europe, kettlebells have been around for decades yet are just starting to increase in popularity in the United States. Ranging in weight from two to a hundred pounds or more, they look like bowling balls with

Spin Rage

The rule at one club where I taught Spinning was that everyone had to sign up for a spot and the bikes went on a first-come, first-served basis. If you weren't in class five minutes after it started, you forfeited your bike and it could be taken by whomever was there.

This system was a mess. There were constant fights between people who had signed up and then shown up late and the people who had taken their bikes as a result. The class sheet was upstairs at the front desk, and people often lied about whether or not they had signed up. For me, as an instructor, it became increasingly tedious and time-consuming to determine who had signed up and who had not, then referee the almost daily altercations, with my having to get off the bike and mediate the arguments when I should have been teaching.

In one case, a couple who had come in late was definitely in the wrong, but they were determined to take the class. The music was loud enough that I couldn't really hear what they were saying, but I could tell that the couple who were now riding were not about to get up and leave. The argument became more and more heated. The investment banking couple had paired off so that the guy was yelling at the guy and the woman was shrieking at the woman. Other class members were alternating between watching the building fracas with interest and looking at me to see what I was going to do.

I decided to ignore them and teach. I stared straight ahead and continued to cue the class.

"Okay. Two-minute climb. Medium-sized hill, out of the saddle. Add some tension so you're about a six out of ten intensity."

handles. They are used for functional full-body movements that engage numerous muscles simultaneously. While they do have "functional" effects, I believe that the majority of kettlebell movements are extremely advanced. They should be done only under the supervision of a qualified instructor and when you have a strong base of strength.

11. **KICKBOXING.** Remember Tae Bo? Kickboxing classes have been around forever and will be around for many decades to come. Delivering one of the few true double-whammy workouts, a kickboxing class blends cardiovascular and strength moves. You will lose weight as well as tone up in a kickboxing class.

So I continued to lead the class, the fight intensified, and I stayed focused on teaching. Out of the corners of my eyes I could see that the investment banker guy was now shaking the handlebars of the other guy's bike and his wife was now face-to-face with the woman, screaming at her to get off. "Takin' Care of Business" pounded through the speakers as I closed my eyes for a moment and pushed up the imaginary hill.

Screams suddenly broke through my visualization, and I opened my eyes. The opening guitar chords of AC/DC's "You Shook Me All Night Long" reverberated off of the sweat-soaked glass walls as I watched the investment banker couple literally dragging the other two off of the bikes by their shirts. They successfully pulled them both off, and a huge shoving match was now taking place just several feet in front of me.

"Hands in third position." I continued to cue the class and looked right through the melee in front of me. Several members outside the studio had noticed the brawl and were now watching with amusement through the glass walls.

The pushing and yelling continued for thirty seconds or so; then it was over. The couple who had been on the bikes to begin with stormed out of the room, and the investment banker couple victoriously mounted their bikes.

"Get ready to go seated. One-minute sprint coming up."

The class continued without missing a beat.

12. **TRX SUSPENSION TRAINING.** Relatively new and created by Fitness Anywhere, TRX uses straps that hang down from the ceiling or a bar with handles on the end. Exercises are performed by placing either the hands or feet in the handles. It is a challenging workout and extremely functional, one that improves total body strength, coordination, and more.

Ask a Trainer: What is Bikram yoga?

Also known as hot yoga, Bikram yoga is a specific type of yoga done in a heated room, around 95 to 100 degrees Fahrenheit. Invented by and named after the yoga master Bikram Choudhury, Bikram yoga involves twenty-six poses, each done twice in a ninety-minute class. My wife took Bikram yoga twice. Each time she came home looking as if she had been beaten up. Some people love the hot element of Bikram yoga; for other people it is too much. One thing is for sure; if you take Bikram yoga, be prepared to sweat.

The more you sweat, the more the scale will move. In other words, if you weigh yourself after a hot yoga class, chances are you will have lost a pound or two. Did you burn 3,500 to 7,000 calories in the class? Nope. It's just water weight.

Yoga

Yoga has exploded in popularity in the last decade or so. Yoga studios are now ubiquitous, and yoga is now an integral part of the gym group exercise curriculum. More and more men are now taking yoga, from the young to those advancing in years.

Yoga is actually a much more complex practice than the average gymgoer realizes. There are many different types, and it is beyond the scope of this book to discuss the specifics of each one. For our purposes the benefits of yoga, in an extremely simplified form, are as follows:

1. Relaxation

2. Flexibility

3. Balance and coordination

4. Body awareness

5. Isometric strength

These are five of the benefits of yoga. I believe that after strength training and cardio, yoga is a third component that rounds out a great fitness plan.

I see more and more men at my club taking yoga. It helps them alleviate back pain. It helps them reconnect their mind to their muscles. Men at my club, the last type of guys you would expect to see in a yoga class, are now hooked. You know that when they are finally taking a class like yoga, there must be something to it.

TIPS FOR TAKING YOGA CLASS

1. **ASK WHAT YOU NEED BEFOREHAND.** Inquire at the front desk what equipment, if any, you need. Quite often yoga only involves a mat, and the gym will often supply them for members. Ask if this is the case. You may also want to bring your own towel for your sweat and possibly a water bottle if the class will be particularly long and/or hot.

2. **INTRODUCE YOURSELF TO YOUR TEACHER.** As when taking any class for the first time, it's a great idea to let the teacher know you are new. This way he or she can help when necessary without drawing unwanted attention your way.

3. **WEAR APPROPRIATE CLOTHING.** Realize that you will be doing moves that require a certain type of clothing. Choose comfortable, tight-fitting bottoms and tops rather than baggy ones. Function trumps fashion. You will be put into a variety of positions that will not be pretty to your fellow classmates if your clothing reveals more than they care to see.

4. **DON'T GET DOWN ON YOURSELF.** Becoming good at yoga takes years of practice. You will most likely be flopping all over the place during your first few classes. This is to be expected. I don't care how athletic you are, taking yoga for the first time is a challenge for everyone. Once again, put your ego aside and accept the challenge. Remember that not only is no one (other than the instructor) really paying attention to you, but yoga people are some of the most kind and caring you will find.

TIPS FOR TAKING SPIN CLASS

1. **ANYONE CAN DO IT.** It doesn't matter what your fitness level is, even if you are a true beginner, you can (and should!) take a spin class. You can go at your own pace. You are in control of how hard and how fast you spin, so there is no need to worry about "keeping up."

2. **PADDED BIKE SHORTS ARE RECOMMENDED.** It's not the workout that's hard when you first start Spinning, it's how sore your butt can be afterward. Invest in a good pair of padded bike shorts before your first class. You will be glad you did.

3. **YOU CAN ALSO BUY A PADDED SEAT COVER.** If you have an especially sensitive rear end, you can also purchase a gel seat cover that you put over the bike seat. This can really help alleviate the initial soreness.

4. **WHAT TO LOOK FOR IN A SPIN INSTRUCTOR.** Real estate is all about location, location, location, and spin class is all about music, music, music. A great instructor who plays horrible music becomes merely a good one. A good instructor who plays great music comes across as phenomenal. Make sense? You need to be motivated throughout the workout, and when it comes to spin it is music first, the personality of the instructor second, and the actual workout a distant third.

5. **SPIN SHOES.** Most group cycling bikes have pedals that have two sides to them. On one side is a cage that you slide your sneaker into, the other has a clip for special bike shoes. You can use either kind. Shoes with clips are similar to the ones cyclists use with the bikes they ride outdoors. The clips make it slightly easier to deliver an efficient pedal stroke, as they pull up on the pedal with each revolution. Do you need spin shoes? No. But many people who spin several times a week tend to buy these shoes over time.

6. **BRING WATER.** You can really work up a sweat while spinning. Bring a water bottle, and drink from it throughout class. You don't want to get dehydrated during your workout.

I taught Spinning for many years, sometimes four or more classes a day. God knows I saw some strange things from my perch atop the spin platform. There was one older gentleman who used to come into my class wearing Bose noise-canceling headphones. I guess he hated my music and just wanted to be a part of the class.

Rule 4: Spin Classes Are as Hard as You Make Them

Once again, in spin class *you* are in charge of both the tension on your bike and how hard you pedal. One person in spin class may burn 600 calories, while another takes it easy and burns 350. It's up to you to challenge yourself. The instructor merely provides the music and the format for the workout. You have to provide the intensity.

The Three Main Categories of Classes

There are essentially three basic types of classes: those that make you sweat, those that make you strong, and those that focus primarily on stretching and relaxation. Of course there is a crossover in many classes, with some involving two or all three of these elements. But each class has a primary focus, which you must identify when designing your overall fitness plan. Do not kid yourself that a mind-body class counts as strength training or a kettlebell class can take the place of your cardio workout. This misunderstanding of the true training effect of a class is one of the major roadblocks to many gymgoers' goal attainment.

Ask a Trainer: What is the Lotte Berk method?

Lotte Berk (1913–2003) was a ballet dancer who developed her own exercise routine with moves similar to those of Pilates and yoga. The precise isometric-type movements involve pulses, holds, and numerous repetitions. Many who take Lotte Berk are looking to develop the proverbial "long and lean" body type. I contend that this class is another self-selecting one: the women who walk through the door are already long and lean. Lotte Berk does not burn significant calories, nor is it strength training in the traditional sense. It is great for building isometric strength and improving flexibility.

Rule 5: The Locker Room Is Not Your Bathroom at Home; Remember That Other People Use It Too

The Locker Room

Oh, do I have some colorful stories about my myriad experiences in gym locker rooms—enough to fill an entire book. But those are for another time. Suffice it to say that the locker room is a huge part of the gym experience. For many people the quality of the locker rooms is even more important than the quality of the exercise equipment. Or the class programming. People want clean, tidy bathrooms. A study actually showed that the number one thing women looked for in their gym was . . . drum roll, please . . .

Cleanliness.

One of the first things I did when I bought my fitness club was to double the maintenance crew's hours as well as their salary. I realize how important it is to have squeaky clean, almost hospital clean, locker rooms. If you are using your gym several times a week or more, you will be spending a significant amount of time in the locker room undressing, using the sauna or steam room, showering, preening, and having conversations with other members. Here are a few guidelines when it comes to locker room etiquette.

1. USE A TOWEL. I am a huge *Seinfeld* fan, and there is one episode that deals with "good naked" and "bad naked." Walking around the locker room in your birthday suit is definitely "bad naked." I am constantly amazed at how many men strut around sans towel, shave sans towel, comb their hair and brush their teeth sans towel. But the one that puts me over the top is the guys who stop and talk to you wearing nothing but a smile. Stop it. Put on a towel. Please.

2. THE HAIR DRYER IS FOR YOUR HAIR. If walking around naked is disturbing, inappropriate use of the hair dryer is downright frightening. For Pete's sake, it's right there in the name. *Hair* dryer. Without painting too graphic a picture, certain gym members use them to dry other parts of their body, often contorting themselves into horrible naked positions in order to do so. Again, not good. Please stop the insanity. Use a towel.

3. NO INAPPROPRIATE GROOMING. For both men and women, no shaving in the steam room or saunas. Most gyms have signs posted to this effect, yet some people ignore them and continue to shave away. Gross. Cut it out.

4. AND WHEN IT COMES TO "MANSCAPING"? I can't believe I am discussing this, but I have had several unpleasant experiences with this practice, including one time when I walked past a row of showers only to witness a guy grooming his privates

while standing mere inches from the glass door. Beyond gross. At the very least, the guy should have had his back to the door. Better yet, put the "manscaping" routine down as something to be done in the privacy of your own home.

5. PUT YOUR TOWELS IN THE HAMPER. Don't leave them on the bench or the floor. As your mother taught you, pick up after yourself.

6. PROTECT YOUR STUFF. Locker room theft is a huge problem in gyms. Management knows it. The bigger the gym membership, the harder it is to control it. I was a victim of this myself many years ago before I learned and began taking added precautions. Not only did a thief steal a significant amount of money from me, he or she had my keys and some documents with my address on it and tried to break into my apartment several days later. Luckily I had changed the locks and ended up with only a partially kicked-in door.

    You need to be aware of this unfortunate fact. One of the main reasons there is so much theft in gym locker rooms is that it's so darn easy. How many times have you opened a locker at your gym only to find it full of someone's stuff? No lock on it and valuable items inside. Do you want to know how easy and lucrative this type of theft is? In Manhattan certain thieves actually pay for a day pass at a gym, $30 and up, just to get access to the locker rooms and start emptying the unlocked lockers.

Trainer Tip: Buy an expensive lock. One with a code, not a key.

Don't buy a cheap lock that a would-be thief can just break off. Invest in a sturdy heavy-duty lock. And get the kind that opens with a code rather than a key. Keys can easily be left at home or lost. If you are afraid you might forget the combination, you can write it in your gym shoe, store it on your phone, program it into your iPod's notes, whatever.

No matter how good your lock is, however, if a bad guy really wants to break in, he will. Never put any truly valuable things inside your locker. Have a Rolex you'd rather die than lose? Don't bring it to the gym. If you have to bring it to the gym, wear it while you work out.

Trainer Tip: Wearing rubber sandals or flip-flops around the locker room and in the shower is a good idea.

Though I am one of the least germphobic people you will ever meet, I have made the mistake of not following this practice and paid the price. You can contract annoying things like plantar warts by walking around barefoot. Cover those feet.

The Pool

I have to be honest, I laugh a little every time someone brags to me that his or her gym has a pool. When I ask how often he or she uses it, it's the rare individual who swims more than a few times a year. Many never use it at all. It's a great selling point for the salespeople at the gym, but only a few members actually take advantage of it.

Because of the space requirement and maintenance costs involved, a pool is not a standard part of most gyms. And if your gym does have a pool, it is quite often small and able to handle only small numbers of swimmers.

But as more and more gyms are also becoming health and wellness centers, pools are becoming more common. Here are a few rules to follow if your gym has a pool.

1. **SHOWER FIRST.** Most fitness centers require you to shower before swimming.

2. **WEAR A SWIM CAP.** Though it's not always mandatory, your wearing a swim cap will be appreciated by your fellow swimmers. Swimming through loose hair is no fun for anyone.

3. **SHARE YOUR LANE.** When the pool is divided into lanes, common courtesy dictates that you share a lane when asked to do so.

4. **STAY ON YOUR SIDE.** When you do share your lane, don't be a hog. Stay on your side. This means no breaststroke or backstroke swimming where your arms or legs encroach on the other swimmer's area.

5. **SWIM IN THE APPROPRIATE LANE.** Often lanes are marked by speed. One lane is for beginner/slower swimmers, others are for intermediate-level swimmers, and still others are for advanced swimmers who can maintain a fast pace. Seed yourself accordingly.

Ask a Trainer. Someone asked me to "swim in circles" when we shared a lane. What does that mean?

"Swimming in circles" is a technique of sharing a lane with two or more swimmers. Instead of staying on one side and swimming back and forth within the same lane lines, you swim down on one side and come back on the other.

The Steam Room versus the Sauna: What Are They For? And What's the Difference?

Think of it like this: the sauna is Arizona, and the steam room is Florida. A sauna is a dry heat, while the steam room gives off wet, humid heat. What are they for? One definition states:

> They both eliminate toxins through sweat, ease joint pain, improve circulation . . . and strengthen the immune system.

I'm not so sure about the validity of any of those claims. What I do know about saunas and steam rooms? That they are darn relaxing. Sometimes there's nothing better after a hard workout than taking a sauna or a steam. That much I will vouch for. So I recommend using either of them to decompress and unwind after a workout. Consider it a reward for a job well done.

Massage: There's the Rub?

I personally love massages. The harder I am training and the closer I get to a race, the more frequently I get them. Supposedly massages:

- Alleviate low back pain
- Enhance immunity by stimulating lymph flow
- Exercise and stretch weak, tight, or atrophied muscles
- Help athletes prepare for, and recover from, strenuous workouts

- Increase joint flexibility
- Lessen depression and anxiety
- Promote tissue regeneration, reducing scar tissue and stretch marks
- Pump oxygen and nutrients into tissues and vital organs, improving circulation
- Reduce spasms and cramping
- Relax and soften injured, tired, and overused muscles
- Release endorphins
- Relieve migraine pain

Some of those claims I believe to be true, such as alleviating back pain and increasing flexibility. Others don't have much science behind them at this time and are therefore anecdotal at best. In fact, when it comes to the claim that massage helps increase circulation, there was a recent study that found just the opposite to be true.

Here's what I do know: Top athletes get massages frequently. Massages feel good. The more sore I am, the better the massage feels. I am therefore going to continue getting massages.

The same study discussed the possible placebo effect of massage. In other words, people believed it was beneficial, therefore it was, regardless of any actual physiological changes in the body. Well, that works for me. If I feel better, I feel better. If you have the time and the money to spend, and especially if you are consistently working out hard, massage can be a great addition to your overall fitness program.

5.

The Gym Is Only Half of the Equation: How to Eat and Diet the Personal Trainer Way

What I love, really love about getting into shape is that it is one of the few things in life I have complete control over. I control both what I take in and what I burn. It may not be easy, but it is that simple. You control what you do or do not put into your mouth and how much you exercise. No one else does.

So get excited. Realize that, yes, you can in fact get into amazing shape once you get honest with yourself and begin to implement lifestyle changes. It won't happen overnight, but if you give it time, I promise it will happen. You can do it. It's up to you.

Rule 1: You Are What You Don't Eat

Let's go back to math again. There are 168 hours in the week. If a client comes to me three times per week, it means that he or she has 165 hours to undo everything we have done. In other words, a crucial component of getting into shape is diet. You need to watch what you eat when you leave the gym, or you are wasting your time and your money. And wasting my time as a trainer for that matter. The saying used to be "You are what you eat"; I say you are what you *don't* eat. We Americans have atrocious eating habits. Abysmal. But you have the power to change that in yourself. You just need to become educated and start making small changes in your eating habits over time. It's just as with exercise, only these changes bring results even faster.

Navigating Nutrition

While the fitness scene has enjoyed its share of myths and fads over the years, it's nothing like what's happening in the nutrition world. From fad diets to the supersizing craze, it seems as though you need serious nutrition know-how to figure out what to eat and what to avoid. But here's the thing: it's all much more simple than you may think. When people ask me for my nutrition philosophy, I take a page from the Godfather of Fitness himself, Jack LaLanne. To wit: "If man makes it, don't eat it." Now, it's easy for him to say that when he's the picture of health, right? Well, it might surprise you to know that LaLanne readily speaks of his background as a kid addicted to sugar. What set him on the path to fitness was the realization, thanks to a nutrition talk he attended, that simple changes in his diet could change his life. They can change yours too—and it isn't nearly as hard as you may think.

Six Food Truths

My motto is "Keep it simple." The following six food truths will get you onto the path toward a healthy lifestyle. Memorize them, write them down, and live them.

1. **BE HONEST WITH YOURSELF.** I can't tell you how many times I've heard the line "I've been exercising like crazy, and I eat everything right, but

I still can't seem to lose weight." So when I see a client sweating it out with me several times a week and he or she is not seeing the results we both want, I start to wonder what's really in that person's refrigerator. Because here's the thing: even though you're telling me that you're eating all the right things, I have a built-in BS detector. I don't need to ask what you eat, I can tell just by looking at you. You know how when you go to the doctor and fill out forms on your health habits, and you may fudge to make yourself seem a little healthier than you really are? Well, busy doctors may not notice, because they're looking for physical conditions, but a trainer isn't so easily fooled. After all, we're in the body business. My role as a trainer is part body mechanic, part coach, part psychologist—and part mind reader. And believe me, trainers have seen it all. So don't be shy about divulging what it is you really snack on at night, in the morning, or in the middle of your workout when I'm not looking. Since I can't be with you 24/7 (although, believe me, sometimes I wish I could put up a video camera in your kitchen), you need to help me out. Don't have a trainer? No sweat—keeping a food journal is a handy gauge for identifying unhealthy patterns so you can alter them.

2. **WHEN IN DOUBT, GO WITHOUT.** The reason your waistline isn't budging may not be *what* you're eating but *how much* you're consuming. And I don't blame you for eating more than you mean to, as it's no secret that our portion sizes are growing right along with our weight. A movie theater is a perfect place to see this madness play out in person: experts at the Center for Science in the Public Interest took movie theaters to task recently when it tested popular movie-menu items and found that a medium popcorn and soda equal 1,610 calories and 60 grams of saturated fat. As much as you might tell yourself, "Oh, I'll only eat half," I'm the first to admit that it can be hard to do once you start munching. So how much is a healthy portion? Use these guidelines as a good starting point for serving sizes:

   - Serving of fish or meat = deck of cards
   - Serving of cheese = size of a domino

- ½ cup of food = size of a baseball
- Fruit or vegetable portion = size of a baseball (note: fruits and vegetables are one area where's it's okay to "overdo" it, but I'm giving this guideline because I think many people actually underestimate their fruit and vegetable intake)

Rule 2: Keep Junk Out of the House

Sounds *so* easy, right? Well, it is. I am just like everyone else: if it's in the house, I'll eat it. I'll eat perfectly all day, then wake up ravenous at 3 A.M., go downstairs, and eat an entire box of Girl Scout cookies. I've been known to break into a can of cake frosting. But if there are no Girl Scout cookies and no frosting in the house, if the worst thing I can eat is an apple, guess what? I'll eat an apple. And I'll enjoy it too. More and more over time.

Don't get me wrong. I still eat Reese's Peanut Butter cups. Jumbo size. And Skittles. And I don't share. (I blame the no sharing on having grown up with five brothers.) I just don't eat them regularly. And I would never keep them in the house. Be a realist: if it's in the house and you're hungry, you'll eat it. Keep the treats out of the house. That's why they call them treats: they're supposed to be for special occasions. Not eaten every day.

3. **EAT REAL FOOD.** This goes back to Jack LaLanne's advice of eating only food that isn't man-made. Think of eating as "clean" as you can, a term bodybuilders use, and you'll automatically be on the route to eating healthfully. Obviously, I don't mean you need to cut out everything that comes with a label, but if you try to follow this rule at least half the time, you're on the right path. I also get a lot of questions about supplements, and here's my advice on that: I believe it's always best to get your vitamins and minerals from actual food. That said, two supplements I do recommend in moderation for men wh are looking to add muscle, in the form of smoothies, are those that contain protein and creatine (which is a naturally occurring amino acid that helps supply energy to your muscles). Food sources of creatine are fish and red meat, but it can be hard to get enough in your daily diet, so that's

why I diverge from my usual "eat real food" philosophy for both of these nutrients, because you can easily get plenty in just a teaspoon, and they're a great addition to a weight training program.

4. **SIP WISELY.** Just as you want to reach for real food rather than supplements, you're better off if you eat real food rather than drinking it. To illustrate this idea, let's take a glass of OJ versus an orange. An eight-ounce glass of juice has 110 calories and less than 1 gram of fiber, while a medium orange has 62 calories and 3 grams of fiber. Which means that not only does the juice take a fraction of the time to "eat," but it has more calories and it's not as filling. The exception to this "don't drink your food" rule is smoothies, which can be a great way to get in your protein, as I mention above, and it's a perfect replenishing snack after a workout.

5. **DON'T GO OVERBOARD WITH SPORTS PRODUCTS.** Ever since the PowerBar was developed in 1983, a slew of sports bars and drinks has sprouted up. There's nothing wrong with these products in and of themselves, as long as you think about the reason they entered the marketplace in the first place: as a way for endurance athletes to eat on the go as they work out. The key word in this sentence is "endurance," which is classified as over sixty minutes. If you're like most people and hit the StairMaster for the standard forty minutes, three times a week, you're better off grabbing some water and a banana. Or if you're in a pinch and use these foods as meal replacements once in a while rather than skipping breakfast, that's great too. As I said, there's nothing wrong with the products in and of themselves, but what you don't want to do is rely on them too much if you're not exercising regularly more than sixty minutes at a stretch.

6. **GET OVER GRAZING.** Grazing became big a few years ago, when the nutrition research began supporting five to six small meals a day. But what then happened was people equated "grazing" with "license to snack all day." This phenomenon has become so widespread that even the satirical newspaper *The Onion* proposed the idea of a "feed bag" that people would attach to their mouths so they can be constantly

eating on the go. Hilarious but scary, right? I'll never forget one client who swore to me that she was eating right but still wasn't losing weight. Well, we happened to be traveling to a race together, and what did she pull out of her bag and ask if I wanted any but a ginormous bag of trail mix—filled with M&M's of course. It was all I needed to know about her diet. (Not that trail mix isn't a good option—in moderation, of course—but there was something about that giant bag and the fact that she was eating it while being idle that answered the question "What the heck is she eating, anyway?") Grazing really means five to six smaller meals each day, not an all-day buffet.

Rule 3: Observe the "One-Cheat" Rule

I look at eating in two ways: in a twenty-four-hour time frame and a seven-day time frame. Within each of those two windows I allow myself one "cheat," or not-so-healthful choice:

1. **TWENTY-FOUR-HOUR RULE:** I eat five to six smaller meals throughout the day. One of those can be a small cheat. So if I have a less-than-healthful breakfast, the rest of the day I eat good meals. If I eat well all day, my final meal can be a little more on the "fun" side.

2. **SEVEN-DAY RULE:** I also give myself one day out of the week to eat less than perfectly. It usually falls on a Friday or Saturday, when I go out to eat with my wife. One day of a little more relaxed eating will not undo a week of good nutrition.

What Do Trainers Eat?

Egg whites. Chicken breasts. Tuna. Fruit. Oatmeal. Salads. Protein shakes.

Repeat. Often.

We trainers like to keep things simple. We stick to what we know. We know how good the above foods will make us look and feel, so we eat them a lot. We generally don't like a whole lot of variation in our diet. Control what you can. You can absolutely control what you put into your mouth.

Whether you like convenient food (not to be confused with convenience-store food) or enjoy cooking, whether you crave variety or prefer to stick to the same foods so you don't have to think about what you eat, I have many quick fixes on page 252 to complete your 24/6. Don't I mean 7? Actually, no—as mentioned above, I truly believe in having one "cheat day" built into your week (most likely on the weekend, when your schedule is usually a little looser anyway). Giving yourself permission to eat whatever you want one day of the week is one of the best things about sticking to a healthful diet—you won't feel as though you're depriving yourself, and you'll be ready to get back on track after one day of eating whatever you want.

Ask a Trainer

Q. What's the most important thing to look at on a food label?

    A. Fat

    B. Fiber

    C. Calories

A. C (calories). Now, I'm not saying fat isn't important (though you shouldn't get more than 30 percent of your calories from fat), and fiber is also an important, filling nutrient (anything over 4 grams is considered high fiber). But when it comes down to it, calories are the most important thing when trying to lose weight. A pound equals 3,500 calories, and it's simple math that you need to burn more calories than you take in. If you take in fewer than you burn, you'll lose weight, and if you take in more than you burn, you'll gain weight. Obviously, you want your calories to be as nourishing as possible (which is why the fat and fiber and vitamin contents shouldn't be ignored), but in the end it all goes back to calories; keep in mind, the average active adult needs 2,000 per day.

Trainer Tip: Eat every two to three hours.

We trainers are always eating. Roughly every two to three hours. Religiously. So should you. You should be eating five to six smaller meals evenly spaced throughout the day. If you eat breakfast (and you should!) at 7 A.M., the day would progress with you eating at 10 A.M., 1 P.M., 4 P.M., and 7 P.M. No bad snacking, just good, high-quality meals.

And please don't tell me you're not hungry and can't possibly eat that often. Right now you're most likely eating three big meals and a handful of "snacks" throughout the day. You're just not aware of it. Every handful, every sip, every bite, taste, and lick of food adds up, my friend.

Rule 4: Food Is *Fuel* First and Foremost

Allow me to get deep for a moment. It's important. Somewhere along the line in history we forgot that the primary purpose of food is to keep us alive. When food became abundant, we suddenly took a 180-degree turn. Now people who eat healthfully are the "outsiders." The exceptions rather than the rule. The "freaks." Eating has become a cause of disease rather than a preventive measure against it. Those who now practice healthful eating and moderation are said not to "enjoy" or "appreciate" food. Those who eat "clean" are labeled negatively, not those who overindulge.

Wrong.

Food is *fuel*. The enjoyment of food should come not from the act of eating it but from how you feel as a result of putting good things into your system. To steal and slightly twist a common phrase, nothing tastes as good as being healthy feels. You put expensive gas into your expensive car, right? Three dollars a gallon or more? Yet people say eating healthfully is expensive. Which is more important? Put cheap gas in, and you get what you pay for. Treat your body like a Ferrari.

Carb Controversy

One of my biggest pet peeves of being a trainer: carbophobes who are convinced that all carbs are bad. So repeat after me: carbs are not the enemy in and of themselves; it's the type of carbs you eat that matter. Carbohydrates are responsible for providing much-needed energy to the body, especially the brain and the nervous system. But there are two types of carbs, simple and complex. Simple carbs are those that are easier for your body to digest, also known as "bad carbs," such as white rice, white bread, and candy. Complex carbs are "good carbs," which make your body work a little harder, such as wheat bread, brown rice, fruit, and vegetables.

Ask a Trainer: How much water should I drink during the day?

My short answer is that we need to drink water throughout the day. Our bodies need to be hydrated to function optimally. I carry a water bottle with me, refilling it several times throughout the day. I don't overdo it. I also sweat tons, almost daily, so I need to replace that water as well.

And let's face it. If you're drinking water, you're not drinking something that's unhealthy, such as soda or some other sugared drink. Water has no calories, it fills you up, and it helps you look and feel great. Drink up.

Rule 5: Don't Waste Your Time Telling Me What You Eat. I *Know* What You Eat. I'm *Looking* at You

This is self-explanatory. Be honest with yourself.

Rule 6: You Are What You Drink—or Don't Drink

So many people drink a huge number of their calories every day. Special coffees, juices, you name it, these drinks often contain a ridiculous number of calories. Don't waste your precious calorie allotment on liquids, especially alcohol. Be very aware of the caloric content of everything you drink. Cutting back on excess liquid calories is one of the fastest ways to shed weight quickly and safely.

How to Beat Your Diet Quick Fixes

REPLACE	WITH
Large muffin and specialty coffee drink	Oatmeal with raisins and coffee with skim milk
Bacon, egg, and cheese on a bagel	Two eggs on whole wheat toast
Regular pasta	Whole wheat pasta
Apple juice	Whole apple
Mid-afternoon candy fix	Protein shake
Potato chip snack	Fresh fruit
Fried appetizer	Vegetable soup

Plan Out Six Small Meals a Day

Meal #1: 7 A.M.: Omelet with vegetables and whole wheat toast

Meal #2: 10 A.M.: Fresh fruit or PowerShake

Meal #3: 1 P.M.: Salad with tuna

Meal #4: 4 P.M.: PowerShake

Meal #5: 7 P.M.: Whole wheat pasta with chicken and vegetables

Meal #6: 9 P.M.: Popcorn

TIP: Try to eat carbohydrate and protein at every meal.

PowerShake Recipe

Makes a simple, highly nutritious, low-calorie meal. Make enough for two servings, and bring one in a shake bottle to work or when you are out on the go. Mix the following ingredients in a blender.

Protein powder

Frozen fruit (strawberries, blueberries, mixed berries, etc.)

1 banana

Water and some ice

1 tablespoon omega fat oil

Rule 7: Read Labels. Closely

Again, go first to calories. Calories, calories, calories. I don't care if an energy bar has 4 "net carbs" if it has hundreds of calories! Even fat grams. It doesn't matter if it's low in fat if it's still chock full of calories. The food industry is incredibly deceiving. Don't be fooled. If it's high in calories, it's trouble.

Shopping List

Berries—frozen or fresh	Raw almonds	Whole wheat pasta
Apples	Unsweetened cocoa	Carrots
Oatmeal	Chicken breasts	Celery
Brown rice	Omega-3 eggs	Almond butter
Whole wheat bread	Lean turkey	Granola
Green tea	Wild salmon	
Low-fat yogurt	Broccoli	

Quick Healthy Eating Tips

1. Eat foods that come without labels (fruit, fresh vegetables, fish, chicken).

2. Stay away from food that has more than five ingredients or comes packaged in a bag (chips, pretzels, candy).

3. Eat your meals sitting down at a table. Avoid eating in your car, in front of the television, or at your computer.

4. Indulge yourself occasionally, but make it a special trip.

5. Eat breakfast.

6. Stay away from fried foods.

7. Keep portion sizes small, and visualize meat more as a side dish than as an entrée.

8. Be adventuresome with fruits and vegetables.

9. Think of food as fuel, not comfort.

10. Keep the temptations out of the house.

Rule 8: It's *Much* Easier to Keep 600 Calories Out of Your Mouth Than It Is to Burn Them Off

It takes the average person about an hour to run off 600 calories. You can drink a Venti White Hot Chocolate with whole milk from Starbucks in a few minutes. Better lace up your running shoes afterward, because that's around 570 calories.

FAQ: What about vitamins? Supplements? What should I take?

Whenever possible, it is best to get your vitamins from real food. But that's not always possible. Why real food? Scientists aren't quite sure why, but getting your vitamin C in a pill is not the same as getting it from an orange. It may have to do with the other compounds in the food as well as other combinations and levels of certain nutrients. Bottom line: it's really complicated.

So we need to eat as healthfully as possible and then try to fill the gaps if we can. People always ask me what supplements I take, and it's not too many things.

1. **MULTIVITAMIN.** I don't eat perfectly. The daily multivitamin gives me what my diet lacks.

2. **GLUCOSAMINE/CHONDROTIN.** Research shows that these two ingredients may have a positive effect on the cartilage in our joints. They might not only help slow the breakdown of cartilage, they might possibly help build new cartilage. Some say yes, some say no way. I say if there's a chance this may be true, I'm willing to risk the money. You can play Lotto; I'll spend my money on Glucosamine and Chondrotin.

3. **OMEGA-3 FATS.** These are good fats. I take them in liquid form, sometimes pills.

I experiment with different supplements every now and again, but those three are my mainstays. I really try to eat the best I can rather than supplementing with pills.

6.

The Twenty-Pack: Your Personal Training Sessions

If I have learned one thing in all my years as a trainer, it's that people really want to know just one thing when it comes to fitness:

What should I do? Just tell me what to do!

So here you go: my most effective workouts, tried-and-true routines that have been tested on hundreds of my clients. Follow them, and you will see results. *Big* results. No two ways about it.

Here is a twenty-pack of training sessions. *Thousands of dollars' worth of workouts.* Each one is different. Some are total-body routines, some are upper-body, some lower-body, some cardio, some core conditioning, and more. I have designed the package so that you can use the sessions in several different ways. If you really want to jump-start your program, go all out and use it as a four-week transformation program. Do the workouts in order, Monday through Friday. They build in complexity and are designed to keep you stimulated mentally as well as physically.

You can also do the workouts out of order. Choose one you feel like doing that day. Remember that you want to let a muscle group rest for at least a day between workouts whenever possible, so try not to do a leg workout one day and another leg workout the next day.

Or you can do five workouts in order for a few weeks, then do the next five workouts in order the next few weeks, and continue that progression. For example, you can do workouts 1 to 5 for three to four weeks, workouts 6 to 10 for the next three to four weeks, and so on.

Just do them. I guarantee they will change your body.

Session 1: Total-Body/Machine Focus

EXERCISE	SETS	REPS
5-minute cardio warm-up, jump rope		
Push-up	1	To failure
Machine chest press	2	12
Machine leg press	2	12
Machine lat pull-down, wide grip	2	12
Machine shoulder press	2	12
Machine leg extension	2	12
Machine triceps extension	2	12
Machine prone leg curl	2	12
Machine biceps curl	2	12
Regular crunch	1	25
Double crunch	1	20
Bicycle crunch	1	60 seconds
Plank	1	30–60 seconds
Push-up	1	To failure

Session 2: Cardio and Core Focus

EXERCISE	SETS	REPS
10 minutes on the treadmill		
Hanging bent-knee crunch	2	20
Straight-arm plank	2	30–60 seconds
Bench crunch	2	20
Seal back extension	2	15
10 minutes on the treadmill		
Hanging bent-knee oblique crunch	2	15 each side
Bird dog	2	10
Oblique crunch	2	20 each side
Cable rope crunch	2	20
10 minutes on the treadmill		

Session 3: Lower-Body Focus

EXERCISE	SETS	REPS
5-minute cardio warm-up, Gauntlet		
Walking lunge	2	20 steps
Smith machine squat	2	12
Smith machine lunge	2	12
Smith machine calf raise	2	12
Dumbbell deadlift	2	12
Bench step-up	2	15
Ball wall sit	2	30–60 seconds
5- to 10-minute cardio cooldown: your choice		

Session 4: Upper-Body Focus, Barbell and Machines

EXERCISE	SETS	REPS
5-minute cardio warm-up, elliptical machine		
Flat-bench barbell bench press	2	12
Machine incline chest press	2	12
Barbell row	2	12
Machine back row	2	12
Machine lateral raise	2	12
Machine shoulder press	2	12
Barbell biceps curl	2	12
Machine biceps curl	2	12
Close-grip barbell bench press	2	12
Machine triceps extension	2	12
Hanging straight-leg raise	2	20
Back extension	2	10
Side plank	2	30 seconds each side
Plank alternating feet	2	30–60 seconds
Push-up	1	To failure

Session 5: Total-Body Focus, Dumbbells

EXERCISE	SETS	REPS
5-minute cardio warm-up, upright bicycle		
Decline bench push-up	1	To failure
Incline dumbbell chest press	2	12
Dumbbell chest fly	2	12
Dumbbell row	2	12
Dumbbell lateral raise	2	12
Dumbbell triceps kickback	2	12
Dumbbell biceps curl	2	12
Dumbbell squat	2	15
Dumbbell bench step-up	2	15
Dumbbell alternating lunge	2	10 each leg
Side crunch	2	20 each side
Two-point plank	2	10 each side
Regular crunch	2	25
Push-up	1	To failure

Session 6: Chest, Shoulders, and Triceps

EXERCISE	SETS	REPS
5-minute cardio warm-up, rowing machine		
Cable chest press	2	12
Machine chest fly	2	12
Incline barbell bench press	2	12
Dumbbell shoulder press	2	12
Cable front raise, straight bar	2	12
Dumbbell rear delt fly	2	12
Cable triceps extension, V-bar	2	12
Dumbbell triceps kickback, single-arm	2	12
Machine-assisted triceps dip	2	10
Side crunch with leg raise	2	20 each side
Rope oblique crunch	2	15 each side
Ball crunch	2	20
Superman	2	10

Session 7: Back and Biceps

EXERCISE	SETS	REPS
5-minute cardio warm-up, treadmill		
Machine-assisted pull-up	2	10
Machine lat pull-down, close grip	2	12
Barbell row	2	12
Machine lat pull-down, supine grip	2	12
Barbell biceps curl	2	12
Cable biceps curl, straight bar	2	12
Preacher bench biceps curl	2	12
Reverse barbell curl	2	12
Crunch	2	25
Two-point side plank	2	30 seconds each side
Ball plank	2	30–60 seconds

Session 8: Legs

EXERCISE	SETS	REPS
5-minute cardio warm-up, jump rope		
Stationary lunge	2	10 each leg
Dumbbell bench step up	2	15 each leg
Ball squat	2	15
Machine leg abduction	2	12
Machine leg adduction	2	12
Barbell deadlift	2	12
Barbell lunge	2	12
Ball hamstring curl	2	15
Dumbbell ball squat	2	12

Session 9: Upper Body/Body Weight

EXERCISE	SETS	REPS
5-minute cardio warm-up, StairMaster		
Push-up	2-3	To failure
Pull-up	2-3	To failure
Incline bench push-up	2-3	To failure
Chin-up	2-3	To failure
Decline bench push-up	2-3	To failure
Dip	2-3	To failure
Push-up	1	To failure
Hanging straight-knee raise	3	20
Plank	1	1-2 min

Session 10: Legs/Unilateral Focus

EXERCISE	SETS	REPS
5-minute cardio warm-up, elliptical machine		
Dumbbell walking lunge	2	20 steps
Single-leg ball squat	2	10
Machine single-leg leg press	2	12
Machine single-leg leg extension	2	12
Machine single-leg prone leg curl	2	12
Machine single-leg calf raise in leg press	2	12
Single-leg dumbbell deadlift	2	10
Bench split jump	2	15

Session 11: Upper-Body/Cable Focus

EXERCISE	SETS	REPS
5-minute cardio warm-up, elliptical machine		
Cable chest press	2	12
Cable chest fly	2	12
Machine lat pull-down, rope	2	12
Machine assisted pull-up	2	10
Cable shoulder lateral raise, handle	2	12
Cable shoulder front raise, straight bar	2	12
Cable triceps extension, straight bar, prone grip	2	12
Cable single-arm bent-over triceps kickback	2	12
Cable biceps curl, straight bar	2	12
Cable single-arm biceps curl	2	12
Cable rope crunch	2	20
Cable rope oblique crunch	2	15 each side

Session 12: Lower-Body Medley

EXERCISE	SETS	REPS
5-minute cardio warm-up, jump rope		
Smith machine squat	2	12
Machine leg press	2	12
Machine seated hamstring curl	2	12
Smith machine lunges	2	12
Machine leg extension	2	12
Machine leg abduction	2	12
Machine leg adduction	2	12
Dumbbell deadlift	2	12
Bench jump	2	15
Ball crunch	2	20
Bench crunch	2	20
Bicycle crunch	2	60 seconds

Session 13: Chest and Back

EXERCISE	SETS	REPS
5-minute cardio warm-up, elliptical machine		
Flat-bench barbell bench press	2	12
Machine lat pull-down, supine grip	2	12
Machine chest fly	2	12
Dumbbell row	2	12
Cable chest press	2	12
Barbell row	2	12
Dumbbell chest fly	2	12
Machine lat pull-down, rope	2	12
Ball push-up	2	10
Plank	2	60 seconds

Session 14: Arms

EXERCISE	SETS	REPS
5-minute cardio warm-up, elliptical machine		
Machine shoulder press	2	12
Dumbbell front and side raise	2	12
Cable front raise, straight bar	2	12
Preacher bench biceps curl	2	12
Barbell biceps curl	2	12
Cable single-arm biceps curl	2	12
Bench dip	2	12
Cable rope skull crusher	2	12
Close-grip barbell bench press	2	12
Hanging straight-knee raise	2	20
Hanging bent-knee raise	2	20
Hanging bent-knee oblique crunch	2	15 each side

Session 15: Legs and Cardio

EXERCISE	SETS	REPS
5-minute cardio warm-up, StairMaster		
Bench crunch	2	15
Side crunch with raised leg	2	15 each side
Bench jump	3	15
Single-leg dumbbell deadlift	2	10
Bench split jump	3	15
Stability ball wall sit	1	60 seconds
Ball hamstring curl	2	15
Ball crunch	2	20
Double crunch	2	15
20 minutes on the StairMaster		

Session 16: Total Body

EXERCISE	SETS	REPS
5-minute cardio warm-up, elliptical machine		
Bicycle crunch	2	60 seconds
Push-up	2	To failure
Ball plank alternating feet	2	60 seconds
Single-leg ball squat	2	10
Cable rope oblique crunch	2	15 each side
Split bench jump	2	15
Superman	2	10
Smith machine barbell squat	2	12
Machine back row	2	12
Machine single-arm biceps curl	2	12
Decline bench push-up	2	To failure
Barbell lunge	2	12
Machine lateral raise	2	12
Machine triceps extension	2	12
Ball wall sit	2	60 seconds

Session 17: Cardio and Core

EXERCISE	SETS	REPS
10 minutes on the treadmill		
Back extension	2	10
Regular crunch	2	25
Hanging straight-knee raise	2	20
Ball plank	2	60 seconds
10 minutes on the Gauntlet		
Straight-arm plank	2	60 seconds
Oblique crunch	2	25 each side
Bird dog	2	10 each side
10 minutes on the rowing machine		
Regular crunch	1	25
Hanging straight-leg raise	1	20
Ball plank	1	60 seconds
Straight-arm plank	2	60 seconds
Oblique crunch	2	25 each side
Bird dog	2	10 each side

Session 18: Total Body

EXERCISE	SETS	REPS
Dumbbell step-up	2	15 each leg
Chin-up	2	To failure
Jump rope	1	2 minutes
Ball squat with dumbbell biceps curl	2	12
Machine assisted pull-up	2	10
Machine single-leg leg press	2	10 each leg
Jump rope	1	2 minutes
Bench crunch	2	20
Incline dumbbell chest press	2	12
Barbell deadlift	2	12
Double crunch	2	20
Cable triceps extension, V-bar	2	12
Jump rope	1	2 minutes
Ball hamstring curl	2	12
Machine single-leg leg extension	2	12 each leg
Regular crunch	3	25

Session 19: Cardio and Core

EXERCISE	SETS	REPS
10 minutes on the stationary bicycle		
Hanging straight-knee raise	2	20
Hanging bent-knee raise	2	20
Hanging bent-knee obliques	2	20
10 minutes on the StairMaster		
Cable rope crunch	2	20
Cable rope oblique crunch	2	20 each side
Plank	2	60 seconds
10 minutes on the treadmill		
Side crunch with leg raise	2	20 each side
Double crunch	2	20
Bicycle crunch	2	60 seconds
Ball crunch	2	20

Session 20: Total-Body/Ball Focus

EXERCISE	SETS	REPS
Ball push-up	2	To failure
Dumbbell ball squat	2	12
Ball plank	2	60 seconds
Ball squat with dumbbell biceps curl	2	12
Ball crunch	2	20
Ball squat with dumbbell shoulder press	2	12
Ball plank alternating feet	2	60 seconds
Single-leg ball squat	2	10
Ball hamstring curl	2	15
Ball wall sit	2	60 seconds

Twenty sessions are not enough? You are hard core! Here are additional workouts that are sure to keep your workouts fresh and the results coming for a long, long time.

The "Sun's Out, Guns Out" Workout

Arms, arms, and more arms. Some days you just want your biceps to be bulging, your triceps to be totally engorged with blood, and your shoulders to feel shredded. This is the workout for just that. Do this routine straight through, two to three times, with little to no rest in between sets.

EXERCISE	SETS	REPS
Barbell biceps curl	1	10
Triceps dip	1	To failure
Dumbbell shoulder press	1	10
Chin-up	1	To failure
Cable triceps extension, V-bar	1	10
Dumbbell front and side raises	1	10
Dumbbell biceps curl	1	10
Cable triceps extension, rope	1	10
Machine shoulder press	1	10

The "Abs"olutely Best Ab Workout

If you really want to flatten your stomach, here is a hard-core workout to harden your midsection. Do this routine two to three times through with little to no rest in between sets.

EXERCISE	SETS	REPS
Regular crunch	1	25
Plank	1	2 minutes
Double crunch	1	25
Side plank	1	60 seconds per side
Bicycle crunch	1	60 seconds
Hanging straight-knee raise	1	25
Cable rope crunch	1	25
Hanging bent-knee raise	1	10 on each side

The Booty Blast Workout

Ladies, want to tone your lower body fast? Here's a quick workout to sculpt your glutes and slim your legs to perfection.

EXERCISE	SETS	REPS
Squat	2–3	15
Machine leg extension	2	12
Bench step-up	2	15
Machine leg press	2	12
Dumbbell deadlift	2	12
Machine prone leg curl	2	12
Dumbbell walking lunge	2	10 steps

The Body-Weight Workout

This is one of my favorites. It's simple, yet extremely effective. Little equipment is needed. But it's not for the faint of heart.

EXERCISE	SETS	REPS
Push-up	2	To failure
Squat	2	15
Dip	2	To failure
Chin-up	2	To failure
Pull-up	2	To failure
Hanging straight-knee raise	2	To failure
Walking lunge	2	10 steps
Plank	2	60 seconds
Bicycle crunch	2	60 seconds
Ball wall sit	2	60 seconds

The "Sing Sing Seven" Prison Workout

Ever notice how guys in prison are generally in pretty great shape? Mostly from workouts done within the confines of their ten-by-ten-foot cells? Here's a workout I use with my clients when I really want to shake things up. No equipment is needed, just a guilty conscience and a desire to suffer. You can do this circuit two or three times through with no rest in between.

EXERCISE	SETS	REPS
Shawshank dumbbell shoulder press	1	To failure
Dead man walking lunge	1	60 seconds
Devil's Island dip	1	To failure
San Quentin wall sit	1	60 seconds
C Block chin-ups	1	To failure
Attica abdominal bicycle crunch	1	To failure
Penitentiary push-up	1	To failure

The Complete Dumbbell Workout

EXERCISE	SETS	REPS
Flat-bench dumbbell chest press	2	12
Single-arm dumbbell row	2	12
Dumbbell shoulder press	2	12
Dumbbell biceps curl	2	12
Dumbbell triceps kickback	2	12
Dumbbells stationary lunge	2	10
Dumbbell squat	2	10
Step-ups with dumbbells	2	10

The Complete Barbell Workout

EXERCISE	SETS	REPS
Flat-bench barbell bench press	2	12
Bent-over barbell row	2	12
Barbell biceps curl	2	12
Close-grip flat-bench press	2	12
Barbell lunge	2	10
Barbell deadlift	2	10

The Perfect 30/30 Cardio and Strength Circuit: Machines

One of my favorite ways to design an hour of training in the gym is thirty minutes of strength training and thirty minutes of cardio. Here is one great program using machines for the strength component that follows that split. For cardio, you get to choose your mode. It can be the treadmill, elliptical machine, bike, whatever. You can also change it around for each ten-minute session, for example doing the StairMaster for the first ten minutes, the elliptical machine for the second ten, and the treadmill for the final ten.

EXERCISE	SETS	REPS
10 minutes of cardio: you choose		10 minutes
Machine chest press	1	10
Machine back row	1	10
Machine shoulder presses	1	10
Machine biceps curl	1	10
Machine triceps extension	1	10
Machine leg press	1	10
Machine leg extension	1	10
Machine leg curl	1	10
10 minutes of cardio: you choose		10 minutes
Repeat strength circuit		
10 minutes of cardio: you choose		10 minutes

The Perfect 30/30 Cardio and Strength Circuit: Dumbbells

Here is another thirty minutes of cardio and thirty minutes of strength training, only this time you will be using dumbbells for the strength circuit.

EXERCISE	SETS	REPS
10 minutes on treadmill		
Incline dumbbell chest press	1	10
Bent-over dumbbell row	1	10
Dumbbell side raises	1	10
Dumbbell triceps kickback	1	10
Dumbbell curl	1	10
Squats with dumbbells	1	10
Dumbbell stationary lunge	1	10 each side
Dumbbell deadlift	1	10
10 minutes on StairMaster		
Repeat strength circuit		
10 minutes on stationary bicycle		

The Perfect 30/30 Cardio and Strength Circuit: Body Weight

Body-weight exercises are great because they are functional and simple, involve minimal to no equipment, and can be done almost anywhere. Yet they are really hard. Here is a circuit involving body-weight exercises that will leave your body screaming for days afterward.

EXERCISE	SETS	REPS
10 minutes of cardio: you choose		
Push-up	1	To failure
Pull-up	1	To failure
Chin-up	1	To failure
Dip	1	To failure
Squat	1	15
Step-up	1	15 each leg
10 minutes of cardio: you choose		
Repeat strength circuit		
10 minutes of cardio: you choose		

The Complete Upper-Body Workout with Cables

EXERCISE	SETS	REPS
Cable chest fly	2–3	12
Cable chest press	2–3	12
Machine lat pull-down, rope	2–3	12
Cable front raise, straight bar	2–3	12
Cable biceps curl, straight bar	2–3	12
Cable single-arm curl	2–3	12
Cable triceps extension, rope	2–3	12
Cable single-arm triceps kickback	2–3	12

The Celebrity Workout

Let's be honest, most celebrities have great bodies to begin with. They are born that way. Many have great genetics. But they also possess one of the most important things when it comes to fitness success: incentive. Huge incentive. When you know you are going to be up on a big movie screen, on television, on stage, or photographed to death, that should give you a strong motivation to want to look your best. Yes, they are being paid to have the perfect body.

I have worked with actors, musicians, models, and the like, people who need to look great for their livelihood. They usually come to me with a month or two to get in "fighting shape"; here is one workout I would use with them. This is to be done with no rest between exercises, repeating the circuit over and over for thirty to sixty minutes or more.

Fit Myth: Workouts by celebrities are the same as workouts designed by a celebrity trainer.

If your car broke down, would you take it to a trained mechanic to get it fixed, someone with years of experience and education, or would you take it to a celebrity? Sure, celebrities generally have great bodies, but, like the people who take Pilates and yoga, the vast majority didn't get them from their exercise routine. And quite often they got it through unhealthy means as well. Remember that our goal is a lifetime of good health and wellness. Yes, we want a great looking-body as well, but you do not have to sacrifice one for the other. The two are not mutually exclusive. That's what *Beat the Gym* is all about, teaching you how to safely achieve the body you want and how to keep it for a lifetime.

Every reality-show "star" with fifteen minutes of fame eventually puts out an exercise video or comes out with a book on diet or exercise. See them for what they are: entertainment.

EXERCISE	SETS	REPS
Jump rope	1	60 seconds
Push-up	1	To failure
Bicycle crunch	1	60 seconds
Bench jump	1	20
Ball squat with dumbbell curl	1	15
Ball squat with shoulder press	1	15
Stairs (running up and down a flight of stairs)	1	60 seconds
Double crunch	1	60 seconds
Bench dip	1	15
Jump rope	1	60 seconds
Single-leg ball squat	1	15 each leg
Bench crunch	1	60 seconds

The Get Huge Workout

Okay. You're a guy [or woman] in your twenties or early thirties. You want to get big. Huge. Here's one workout routine that will help to get that way. It's a three-day cycle, hitting each body part twice a week.

MONDAY	TUESDAY	WEDNESDAY	THURSDAY	FRIDAY	SATURDAY	SUNDAY
Chest, shoulders, triceps	Back, biceps	Legs	Chest, shoulders, triceps	Back, biceps	Legs	REST

Monday and Thursday

EXERCISE	SETS	REPS
Barbell bench press	3	10
Incline dumbbell chest press	3	10
Flat-bench dumbbell chest press	3	10
Dumbbell shoulder press	3	10
Dumbbell front raise	3	10
Dumbbell lateral raise	3	10
Dip	3	To failure
Cable triceps extension, V-bar	3	10
Single-arm dumbbell triceps kickback	3	10
Push-up	1	To failure

Tuesday and Friday

EXERCISE	SETS	REPS
Pull-up	3	To failure
Machine lat pull-down	3	10
Single-arm dumbbell row	3	10
Chin-up	3	To failure
Barbell biceps curl	3	10
Dumbbell biceps curl	3	10
Dip	3	To failure
Cable triceps extension, V-bar	3	10
Single-arm dumbbell triceps kickback	3	10
Push-up	1	To failure

Wednesday and Saturday

EXERCISE	SETS	REPS
Smith machine barbell squat	3	10
Machine leg press	3	10
Smith machine lunge	3	10
Machine leg extension	3	10
Machine prone leg curl	3	10
Barbell deadlift	3	10
Smith machine calf raise	3	10
Machine calf raise in leg press	3	10

The 20-Minute Total Body Blast

Even if you only have twenty minutes to exercise, you can still get a great workout in. Here's a fat-blasting routine you can do when time is tight.

EXERCISE	SETS	REPS
Jumping jacks	1	60 seconds
Push-up	2	To failure
Regular crunch	1	25
Ball squat with dumbbell shoulder press	1	12
Ball squat with dumbbell biceps curl	1	12
Dumbbell row	1	12
Dumbbell triceps kickback	1	12
Dumbbell squat	1	10
Push-up	1	To failure
Bicycle crunch	1	60 seconds
Plank	1	60 seconds

The 60-Second Circuit

One minute per exercise. Ten exercises. Do this circuit two to six times through, or until you have to crawl out of the gym on your hands and knees.

EXERCISE	SETS	REPS
Jump rope	1	60 seconds
Squat	1	60 seconds
Bicycle crunch	1	60 seconds
Push up	1	60 seconds
Jumping jacks	1	60 seconds
Walking lunge	1	60 seconds
Plank	1	60 seconds
Bench dip	1	60 seconds
Bench jump	1	60 seconds
Double crunch	1	60 seconds

7.

I've Got It, Now How Do I Keep It?: Maintaining Your Fitness and Staying Motivated

One of the hardest concepts to get across is that, yes, eventually your consistent hard work will pay off. Not only will it pay off in terms of seeing results, it will also pay off in a much more profound way: you will actually be able to do less—much less—and still continue to get results.

That's right: do *less* work and still look great.

I know it's hard, at the beginning, to fathom that you'll eventually be able to work out less. I promise you will. It is going to get easier. But you have to earn it first.

I used to work out for several hours a day back when I was starting out as a trainer. Today my gym workout is often a quick twenty-minute full-body workout. With light weights. Including abs. What I want you to realize is that you can do this too. You too can reach this so-called maintenance phase. If you follow the methodology outlined in this book, you'll be there before you know it. And how great it is when you attain it! It is a huge reward for all your hard work.

The Maintenance Phase: For Many of Us, This Is a Dream That We Can't Picture Being a Reality

It does take a while before you enter this maintenance phase. How long? It depends on how hard and how consistently you work out. For the vast majority of exercisers it happens later in life, after they've spent some serious time in the gym. If you've worked your butt off consistently since you were a teenager, it can happen in your thirties.

Not only *can* you exercise less once you enter the maintenance phase of your training, you *should* exercise less. Many injuries occur because people continue to do the same workouts and try to use the same weight they have been using for years. As you get older, you must modify your program. Your body becomes much less resilient as you get older. You don't bounce back or recover as fast. Your body isn't as forgiving. Think quality over quantity.

The "ADD" Workout

One workout I love to do now I call the "ADD" Workout. Referring to "attention deficit disorder," it is basically a full-body workout with no structure whatsoever. Those of you who have reached the maintenance phase can do this workout frequently; those of you who are not there yet can do it once a month or so, just to shake things up.

It's very simple: just go into the gym and do whatever the heck you feel like doing. One set of leg extensions, a set of chin-ups, sixty seconds of the plank, twenty-five push-ups, rope triceps press-downs, two minutes of jumping rope, and so on. Don't think. Don't you dare wait for a piece of equipment. Just keep moving, doing one set per exercise. You can do more than one set of a particular exercise, just not in a row.

I'd outline an ADD Workout for you here, but that would go against the very definition of it. You make it up. No two ADD Workouts should ever be the same.

Sample Maintenance Week

MONDAY	TUESDAY	WEDNESDAY	THURSDAY	FRIDAY	SATURDAY	SUNDAY
30 minutes full body	30–60 minutes cardio	30 minutes full body	30 minutes full body or REST	30–60 minutes cardio	30 minutes full body	REST

Rebalancing Your Exercise Portfolio

My dad works in finance. I have five brothers. All of them work in finance. I know very little about finance, but one concept I am familiar with is the rebalancing of one's portfolio as we age. There is a perfect correlation between fitness and finance when it comes to this concept of changing your "portfolio" as you grow older.

In finance, we tend to have riskier investments when we are younger. With each subsequent decade we decrease the percentage of risky investments; adding in more stable, tried-and-true products

We need to do exactly the same thing with our exercise programs.

As we age, we have to pull back a little when it comes to our workouts, take out the riskier moves. Find the exercises that have the least chance of injury with the highest chance of reward. I designed workouts recently for a *Men's Journal* article that had programs for each decade of your life, exercise routines you should do while in your twenties, thirties, forties, and so on. With each decade comes a shift in the focus and type of exercises. You need to modify your workouts accordingly as well.

Don't misunderstand me. I'm not saying you have to throw in the towel or give in to getting older. I am the first to say that age is merely a number. I am forty-one and still getting faster. My personal best marathon and Ironman times are in my future, not my past. But even I have made certain modifications to my cardio and strength training routines over the years. Here are a few guidelines that you can follow as well.

1. **GO LIGHTER.** This is so obvious, yet so difficult to follow. We need to lift lighter weights as we grow older. Your focus should be on continuing to challenge the muscles during each exercise rather than worrying about how much weight you are lifting. Once again, let the glory days go. Lift with your head, not your ego.

2. **TRY NOT TO RUN TWO DAYS IN A ROW.** Unless you are a serious runner, take a day off in between runs whenever possible. Running on Monday, Wednesday, Friday, and Sunday is so much easier on your body than running on four consecutive days. You can still challenge your body; just give it a little more time to recover.

3. **BE CAREFUL WITH EXPLOSIVE MOVEMENTS.** Movements such as plyometrics and sprints should be done judiciously as we age. Any sudden starts and stops carry an increased risk of injury. Notice I didn't say you can't do them, just know your limits.

4. **DO LONGER WARM-UPS.** Before engaging in any type of exercise, especially higher-intensity activities, be sure to do a nice long warm-up, some kind of low-intensity full-body movement that gets the blood flowing and increases your core temperature. So many injuries that occur during tennis, basketball, and similar activities can be avoided by warming up sufficiently beforehand.

5. **USE DUMBBELLS INSTEAD OF BARBELLS.** You will rarely see me do a bench press with a barbell today. Barbells afford less freedom of movement, which can result in injury, especially to the shoulder joint. Dumbbells are less fixed and therefore place less strain on certain parts of the body, lessening the likelihood of injury.

Stay Motivated, Stay Strong

My job is not only to get clients into the best shape of their lives, it is also to educate them so that they can maintain it on their own. There comes a time in the trainer/client relationship when we must part ways. As sad as ending the relationship may be, I take great pride in knowing that my clients leave with the knowledge, experience, and techniques to work out anytime, anywhere.

You have now read this book. You may have tried a workout or two already. You possess a newfound enthusiasm and excitement for what your fitness future may bring. You now have all the tools you need to transform your body and transform your life.

Go get what is yours. Bring out the best you.

Beyond the Gym

I will always go to the gym. Forever. Whether it's my own club or a gym while I'm traveling, I will forever crave the endorphin high from a sweaty hour of cardio, the pump from the blood cascading to my muscles after a hard arm workout, the stress release that comes only after stressing the body through hard, deliberate exercise. I love it.

But just as you must mix up your strength training and cardio routines, you also must add variation to your fitness plan as a whole. You need to continue to explore new areas of the fitness world, take on challenges that seem just out of reach. Petrified of swimming? Sign up for a triathlon. Deathly afraid of heights? Climb a mountain. Push your limits. Take yourself just outside your comfort zone. Stay there awhile. Life is short, and we must all appreciate our health while we have it. Never, ever take it for granted.

Acknowledgments

Ever since I was ten years old I have loved to write. The opportunity that writing books affords me, to combine my passions of writing and fitness while reaching thousands of people around the world, is truly humbling.

First and foremost, thank you to William Morrow and HarperCollins for publishing *Beat the Gym*. Special thanks to my incredible editor, Matthew Benjamin, who waited patiently and never once chastised me as I missed deadline after deadline. Your unending patience was only surpassed by your ability to arrange my crazy thoughts and ideas. Thank you.

Thank you to my literary agent extraordinaire, Lauren Galit. To think what we started with and what we ended up with is staggering. You made the process painless, educational, and even fun. I look forward to working with you for many years to come.

Thank you to Megan McMorris, prolific writer and all-around great person. What were we working on again? Thank you for your expertise and unending support.

Thank you to my "Ari," agent Topher DesPres at the Wilhelmina Agency. To think what we have accomplished in such a short time is incredible. Many big things to come.

Thank you to PR gurus Melissa McNeese and Leslie McClure. You got all of this started and I am forever grateful.

Finally, thank you to my amazing wife, Philippa. None of this would have happened without you.

Special thanks to Tricia Nisenson, Trish Daly, William Simpson, Brady Quinn, Lucy Danziger, Tamilee Webb, Joanna Graf, and Andy Dover.

Choosing
a Personal Trainer

B*eat the Gym* is designed to be your personal trainer, but if you want to try out the real thing, you should. I have spent years helping people out, and there are wonderful trainers. It is a significant investment of money as well as time. You want to make sure that you get what you are paying for. You also want to make sure you choose someone who won't hurt you. Realize that the number of trainers has increased exponentially over the past decade. Anyone, and I mean anyone, can call himself a personal trainer. As someone who has worked as a trainer in every type of gym imaginable, alongside every type of trainer imaginable, here are my rules for finding the right training for you.

Rule 1: Not All Trainers Are Created Equal

There are four basic criteria you want to use when considering hiring a personal trainer:

1. Certifications
2. Experience
3. Methodology
4. Lifestyle

Certifications

Many trainers have a bunch of letters after their name on their business card. Some denote a master's degree, while others represent numerous different fitness certifications. While you really want work with a trainer who is certified and the more certifications the better, you need to know which ones are the best ones and which ones don't count for much.

There are literally dozens of fitness certifications out there. They are not all created equal by any stretch of the imagination. Some are much better than others. In fact, it would surprise most people to learn how little fitness knowledge is required to pass most fitness certifications. Few, if any, require any practical hands-on component. Some can be purchased right over the Internet; others require one- or two-day workshops followed by a test at the end.

A trainer who has an undergraduate and/or graduate degree in exercise science or a related field is a great start. They will have a great foundation of knowledge about how the human body works. Add certifications on top of that, and you have the makings of a great trainer.

Just because a trainer looks great does not mean he is qualified. And yes, there are many trainers working in gyms who have no certifications whatsoever. It is an unfortunate fact that many people get hurt by working with trainers who put them through inappropriate routines.

The Four Certifications to Look For

The four certifications that are considered the best in the business are the National Strength and Conditioning Association's Certified Strength and Conditioning Specialist (NSCA-CSCS) and those provided by the American College of Sports Medicine (ACSM), the National Academy of Sports Medicine (NASM), and the American Council on Exercise (ACE). Trainers who hold one or more of these certifications have a certain understanding of anatomy, kinesiology, biomechanics, and the body's energy systems.

Rule 2: There Is No Law That Trainers Need to Be Certified. In Any State

That goes for personal training certifications and even CPR. Just because the trainers in your gym are walking around in a uniform with a name tag does not mean they have a certification. Some gyms today require new trainers to hold at least one certification when they are hired.

Some.

Ask your potential trainer what organizations he or she has been certified by. Don't just take his or her word for it, either. Ask to see his or her certification card.

TOP CERTIFICATIONS

1. **ACSM:** American College of Sports Medicine
2. **NSCA:** National Strength and Conditioning Association
3. **ACE:** American Council on Exercise
4. **NASM:** National Academy of Sports Medicine

Experience

Rule 3: A Good Trainer Has Years of Experience

Certification alone is not enough to make a qualified trainer. Most certifications are knowledge- and not practice-based. In other words, you can't become a great trainer by book knowledge alone. A trainer needs experience. Ideally, he or she has been working in the industry for a while. The longer, the better. You definitely don't want to be a new trainer's guinea pig, the person on whom he will make mistakes and ultimately learn from. The cost can be high. You want a trainer who has worked with as diverse a population as possible, someone who has refined his technique and methodology through years of experience in the gym. Great trainers are made, not born.

Along with experience is each trainer's specialty. Are you a runner who wants to train for a marathon? Then ideally you would hire a trainer who has experience working with runners. Want to learn to box? Find a trainer who knows the most about boxing. Be wary of trainers who seem to be jacks-of-all-trades. Yes, a qualified trainer should be able to work with a wide variety of people, but combining certifications and experience with a specific specialty is the best of all possible worlds.

Methodology

Rule 4: Observe Your Trainer in Action

The third criterion in selecting a trainer is her personal methodology. How does she train her clients? Observe her in action. See exactly how she spends the hour with her clients. Does she give her undivided attention, or is she staring off into space? Does she talk incessantly, using the hour as her personal therapy session? You can learn a great deal about a trainer by just watching her from afar.

If you have been a member of your gym for a while, you already have a pretty good idea of what the trainers are like: what type of clientele they have, the types of workouts they utilize, and their professionalism at work. Do they do the same exact workout with each and every client? This is a big red flag. As discussed earlier, no one workout works for everyone. Yes, there are certain exercises that are great and benefit many clients, but there is no one workout that should be done by all. Before you do one session with a trainer, watch him or her in action for at least a few days.

Lifestyle

Rule 5: Don't Choose an Unfit Trainer

At its simplest, lifestyle can stand for how the trainer looks. Is he or she in shape? Call me crazy, but I firmly believe that fitness professionals need to be in shape. A trainer who is out of shape is analogous to a financial planner who is in debt. Both can work in their respective industries, but only after they have been successful at what they plan to teach people how to do.

If the trainer is in shape, then take things one step further. Does he or she have the body that *you* aspire to having? A qualified trainer will be able to sculpt any type of body you desire, but it's much better if he possesses the kind you are looking for. It will serve to inspire and motivate you. He will have a deeper understanding on how to help you achieve the body you want. If you want a long, lean body like a dancer, try to find a trainer who has achieved that look. If you want quads and biceps like Arnold, seek out a similarly sculpted trainer.

Is it essential to work out with a trainer who possesses your dream body? No. But it helps a lot.

Rule 6: Good Trainers Do Much More than Serve as "Appointment Holders" at the Gym

Personal trainers wear a number of hats, the three most important being:

1. Designing custom, periodized workouts tailored specifically to you

2. Ensuring that you do each exercise with proper form, maximizing your results and minimizing the likelihood of injury

3. Pushing you to work harder than you would on your own

Building a Home Gym

I have designed many home gyms for clients over the years, costing anywhere from $100 to $50,000 and more. The great news is that you do not have to spend a lot of money to create a fantastic home gym. In fact, the cost of a home gym is quite often inversely proportional to the amount of usage it gets. Here are the three basic elements you need to create your own private workout space:

1. **A MAT.** A cushioned mat that you can put down on the floor to do abdominal exercises, stretching, push-ups, and so on. Shouldn't cost much at all. The thicker the mat, the pricier it gets.

2. **SEVERAL SETS OF DUMBBELLS.** Dumbbells are inexpensive, yet you can do an infinite number of exercises with them. Get two to three sets to start: a light, medium, and heavy set. For most women that means five

pounds, eight pounds, and ten pounds. Men can get started with tens, fifteens, and twenty-fives.

3. **A STABILITY BALL.** A stability ball is one of the greatest pieces of home exercise equipment. It has many great qualities, including:

    a. It can serve as your bench without being heavy or expensive and permanently taking up part of a room.

    b. You can move it around easily and deflate it when you want to store it.

    c. You can do leg, abdominal, and upper-body exercises with it, stretch on it, and much, much more.

    d. You'll never have buyer's remorse after buying one.

Trainer Tip: Stability balls come in different sizes based on your height.

Many people just go into a store, pick up a stability ball, and buy it. You need to know that there are different sizes:

YOUR HEIGHT	BALL SIZE (CM)	BALL SIZE (IN.)
Under 5'	45	17
5'–5'7"	55	21
5'8"–6'2"	65	25
Over 6'3"	75	29

These sizes are general, not set in stone. Different leg lengths can change what size ball certain people need. A simple rule is that when you are sitting on the ball your legs should be at a ninety-degree right angle, with your thighs parallel to the floor.

Other Items to Add to Your Home Gym

A mat, dumbbells, and a stability ball will get you started on your way to maintaining your workouts when you can't get to the gym. Here are a few additional things that you can add to your home exercise arsenal.

1. **A JUMP ROPE.** It's inexpensive and easy to store. You can jump rope anywhere, even outside. I know, you're probably not so good at it. Well, that's even better. The worse at it you are, the more calories you'll burn. Even if you are good at jumping rope, it's one of the best ways to burn calories fast.

2. **DVDS.** Workout DVDs are ridiculously cheap today. There are DVDs for every conceivable exercise type, so you can get a bunch of what you like. Pilates, yoga, tai chi? Yogilates? Beach Booty? Some remastered Jane Fonda, perhaps? DVDs are great in that you have a set routine to follow and hopefully an instructor who demonstrates proper form. You can also rotate the DVDs to keep you interested as well as mixing up your workouts.

3. **ONE PIECE OF CARDIO EQUIPMENT.** Now we're getting pricier, but if you think you'll do some cardio at home, by all means invest in a good piece of cardiovascular equipment. Choose the piece that you think you will use the most. For many people nowadays it's an elliptical trainer first, with a treadmill coming in second. But it could be a stationary bike, a rower, a StairMaster, whatever you think you will really use. Remember that your heart is a muscle, the most important muscle, and you need to exercise it. I realize that elliptical trainers and treadmills can get expensive, but remember that you are investing in your health. What better to spend your money on?

Index

chest
- Get Huge Workout and, 273–74
- personal training sessions for, 259, 262, 273–74
- regions of body and, 170
- *See also specific exercise*

chest fly, 60, 89, 174, 258, 259, 261, 262, 271

chest press
- barbell, 86, 87
- cable, 135, 259, 261, 262, 271
- dumbbell, 86, 90, 184, 258, 264, 268, 270, 273
- flat-bench, 86, 90, 268, 273
- machine, 55, 61, 256, 258, 269
- strength training and, 76, 135
- tweaks to increase effectiveness of, 174

chin-ups, 117, 172, 260, 264, 266, 267, 269, 271, 274

chondroitin, 254

circuit training, 39, 76–77, 170

classes, group exercise, 223–42
- appropriate clothes for, 229, 235
- arriving late to, 228
- avoiding, 227–28
- benefits of, 224–25
- burn out and, 227
- categories of, 237
- descriptions of, 230–35
- etiquette for, 228–29
- fear of, 223–24, 227–28
- fees for, 5
- fitness plan and, 225, 237
- gender and, 224, 227
- instructors of, 227
- leaving early from, 228
- mistakes to avoid when taking, 227–28
- "newbies" in, 223–24
- place in, 228
- purpose of, 223
- rules about, 225–26, 229
- self-consciousness in, 224
- singing and shouting in, 228, 229
- as substitute for fitness training, 225–26
- types of, 226
- variation in, 226, 227
- *See also type of class*

cleanliness, 7–8, 238

clothes
- for classes, 229, 235
- in locker rooms, 238

commercial workout, cardio, 38

compound exercises, 171–72

contracts, 3–4

cooldown, cardio, 39, 257

core conditioning classes, 230–31

core exercises, 150–67
- breathing during, 219
- fun "toys" for, 195
- group exercise classes for, 230–31
- how often to do, 216
- importance of, 150–51
- personal training sessions for, 257, 263, 264
- rules about, 168
- weight belts and, 205
- *See also* abdominals; glutes; lower back; *type of exercise or specific exercise*

creatine, 246–47

crunches
- Attica abdominal bicycle, 268
- ball, 156, 259, 261, 264, 265
- bench, 162, 257, 261, 264, 273
- bicycle, 163, 185, 214, 217, 256, 261, 263, 264, 266, 267, 268, 273, 275
- cables and, 133–34, 257, 261, 264, 266
- as core exercises, 156–63
- don't do, 186
- dos and don'ts of, 219
- double, 161, 189–90, 256, 264, 266, 273, 275
- flexing spine during, 212
- hands across chest, 157, 218
- hands behind, 218
- hanging bent-knee, 257, 262
- how often to do, 216
- importance of doing, 188
- oblique, 134, 158, 257, 259, 261, 262, 263, 264
- old-school, 186
- personal training sessions and, 256, 257, 258, 259, 263, 264, 266, 275
- reverse, 214
- rope, 133, 134, 188, 257, 259, 261, 264, 266
- side, 159, 160, 258, 259, 264
- spot reduction and, 182
- strength training and, 133–34
- time during workouts devoted to, 188
- tips for doing, 218, 219, 220
- weights and, 219
- workout partners and, 169

curls
    barbell reverse, 95, 259
    cable single-arm, 271
    dumbbell, 270, 273
    squats with, 273
    See also type of curl
cycling, group, 225

Hamstrings (*cont.*)

See also hamstring curls

health, and fitness, 10

heart rate, 14–15, 20, 23, 26, 31, 42, 76, 226

hills, cardio machines and, 39

hip abduction exercises, 182

home gyms, 291–93

human growth hormone, 206

I

infomercial, television, 182

insanity classes, 226

IntenSati, 226

intensity

age and, 280

cardiovascular health and, 18–19, 216

excuses trainers hear about, 17

on NordicTrack, 31

plyometrics and, 199

rules about, 187

stationary bikes and, 23, 26

on treadmills, 20

of warm-up, 37

of workouts, 12–13, 15, 17, 280

intervals, 39

isolation exercises, 171, 172

isometric exercises, 173, 231, 234, 237

isotonic exercises, 173

IT (iliotibial) band, 195

J

jogging, 12, 19

joints, 19, 22, 28, 37

See also compound exercises

jump rope, 41, 226, 256, 260, 261, 264, 273, 275, 293

jumping jacks, 41, 203, 275

jumps

bench, 130, 131, 199, 260, 261, 263, 273, 275

plyometrics and, 199

junk food, 246

K

kettlebells, 226, 231–32

kickback. See triceps kickback

kickboxing, 226, 232–33

knee raise

hanging bent-, 151, 262, 264, 266

hanging straight-, 153, 260, 262, 263, 264, 266, 267

knees

core exercises for, 151, 153

leg extensions and, 178

"locking out" of, 182

myths about, 205

See also knee raise

L

lactic acid, 221

LaLanne, Jack, 244, 246

lateral exercises

"tweaks" to increase effectiveness of, 175

See also lateral pull-downs; lateral raise

lateral pull-downs

behind the head, 193–94

to chest, 194

exercises to avoid and, 193–94

grips for, 68, 69, 70, 256, 259, 262

machine, 68, 69, 70, 71, 256, 259, 261, 262, 271, 274

rope, 71, 261, 271

wide bar, 68, 70

lateral raise

cable shoulder, 140, 261

dumbbell, 258, 273

machine, 48, 258, 263

laundry service, 10

leg abduction, machine, 53, 260, 261

leg adduction, machine, 54, 260, 261

leg curls

machine, 49, 50, 62, 256, 267, 269, 274

machine single-leg prone, 50, 260

prone, 49, 50, 256, 260, 267, 274

seated, 62

single-leg, 50

strength circuit and, 77

leg extension

"locking out your knees" and, 182

machine, 51, 52, 178, 183, 256, 260, 261, 264, 267, 269, 274

physical therapy and, 178

single-leg, 52, 260, 264

strength circuit and, 77

leg lifts

hanging, 214

straight, 189

leg press

calf raise in, 260, 274

as compound exercise, 172

"locking out your knees" and, 182

machine, 44, 56, 57, 58, 59, 256, 260, 261, 264, 267, 269, 274

single-leg, 57, 260, 264

speed of, 201

warm-ups *(cont.)*
    aging and, 280
    cardio, 36–37, 256, 257, 258,
        259, 260, 261, 262, 263
    "dynamic," 36–37
    favorite ways to do, 41
    intensity of, 37
    length of, 36–37
    personal training sessions
        and, 256, 257, 258, 259,
        260, 261, 262, 263
    plyometrics and, 199
    stretching as, 36–37
water, drinking, 236, 251
websites: checking out gym, 6
weight, of bars, 188, 210
weight belts: myths about, 205
weight, body
    classes helping with, 232
    diet and, 243–54
    elliptical trainers and, 29
    excuses trainers hear about,
        16–17
    "fat-burning" prog1rams
        and, 12–13
    joints and, 22
    losing, 249
    mathematics of calories and,
        34
    and running and, 12, 22, 35
    walking and, 35
    yoga and pilates and, 42
    See also body-weight
        exercises
weight vests, 33
weights
    Ask a Trainer about, 177

bulking up and, 168
changing type of, 185
crunches and, 219
drop sets with, 207–8
egos and lifting, 201
endurance and, 168
etiquette concerning, 204
gender and, 168
grips when lifting, 184
how often to lift, 177
increasing, 187
lifting, 39, 45, 168, 177,
    184
pyramid sets with, 208
rules about lifting, 168
too much, 176, 187
total body conditioning
    classes and, 231
tricks for body building
    and, 200
tweaks to increase
    effectiveness of, 174, 175
wrong way to lift, 45
wheels, 198
women
    body bars and, 188
    classes for, 224
    dumbbells in home gym for,
        291–92
    group exercise classes and,
        227
    myths about strength
        training and, 206
    See also gender
woo-ing, 228, 229
"working in," 203, 204

workouts
    alternating routines during,
        177
    Ask a Trainer about, 177
    celebrity, 272–73
    division of time during, 188,
        211
    exercises to omit from,
        189–94
    exercises you hate and, 205
    groups for, 169
    increasing exercise arsenal
        during, 169
    intensity of, 12–13, 15
    in magazines, 206
    maximizing, 40
    order of exercises in, 184
    partners for, 168–70
    soreness after, 221
    splitting up, 207, 269
    start of, 205
    stretching after, 37
    variation in, 184, 203, 225,
        226, 227, 281
    See also specific workout

Y

yelling/shouting, 204, 228
yoga, 42, 173, 225, 226, 230,
    234–35
    See also yogilates
yogilates, 226, 231

Z

Zumba, 226, 230